BEAUTY
HACKS

BEAUTY HACKS

Copyright © Summersdale Publishers Ltd, 2017

Illustrations by Kostiantyn Fedorov

With research by Agatha Russell

An Hachette UK Company
www.hachette.co.uk

Summersdale Publishers Ltd
Part of Octopus Publishing Group Limited
Carmelite House
50 Victoria Embankment
LONDON
EC4Y 0DZ
UK

www.summersdale.com

Printed and bound in Croatia

ISBN: 978-1-84953-574-8

BEAUTY HACKS

Make-Up Cheats, Skincare Tricks and Styling Tips

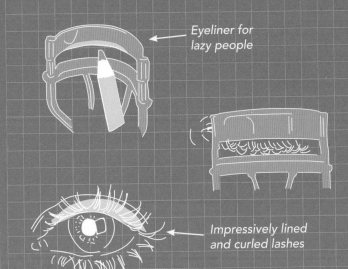

Eyeliner for lazy people

Impressively lined and curled lashes

Aggie Robertson

Over **130** amazing hacks inside!

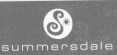

summersdale

DISCLAIMER

Neither the author nor the publisher can be held responsible for any loss or claim arising out of the use, or misuse, of the suggestions made herein. Always test a small amount of any home-made concoctions first, either on the back of your hand or behind your ear, to check for allergic reactions. Consult your doctor before embarking on any new exercise programme or diet.

CONTENTS

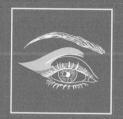
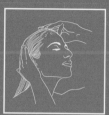
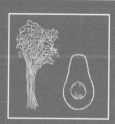
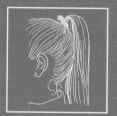
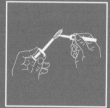
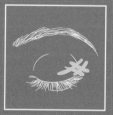
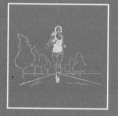
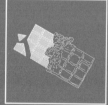
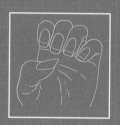
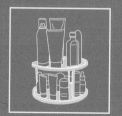
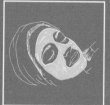
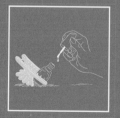

INTRODUCTION

Welcome to *Beauty Hacks,* the must-have book for anyone who wants to master the art of being effortlessly beautiful. Whether you are an out-and-out beauty expert or someone who just wants to look great on the go without breaking the bank, this book is full of tips and tricks for life's beauty dilemmas. You'll be able to carry on strutting your stuff in true style while saving time, money and effort; these hacks are so clever that they may even inspire you to try out some new looks.

So, if your favourite nail polish keeps going sticky, an outbreak of blackheads has left you feeling like a complete and utter recluse or you think you've got the worst 'smoky eye' technique, don't panic. We've got it covered here with our top tips and easy fixes to set you straight – read on to discover the beauty secrets you won't be able to live without.

MAKE-UP TRICKS

Make-up shouldn't need to come with a detailed blueprint: it's simple, and with these tips it will be a cinch. Girls-on-the-go need fast, feature-enhancing tips that will make them look fantastic but without all the work.

ICE CUBE PRIMER

Before you even start applying make-up, this simple trick is the perfect way to prime your skin. Wrap an ice cube up in a thin flannel or thick, soft tissue (you don't want it to stick to your skin), and rub gently over your face, concentrating on areas where your pores are most visible. The cold ice will close up pores and minimise their appearance under make-up for a smooth, long-lasting effect.

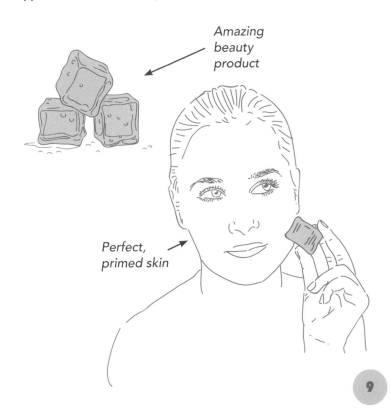

Amazing beauty product

Perfect, primed skin

HEATED CURLERS

Just like the hair on your head, eyelash curls set quicker and more effectively with the help of heat. Take your lash curlers and heat them with a hairdryer for no more than 10 seconds. Wait a few seconds for them to cool slightly, then check with your finger that they are warm but not hot. Then place them over your eyelashes and curl like you normally would. Finally apply mascara for wide, beautiful lashes - no false ones needed!

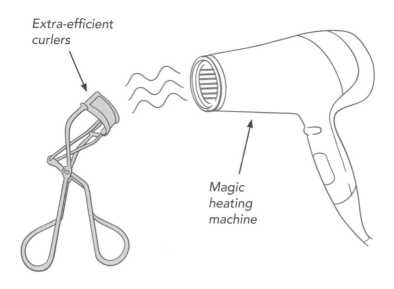

Extra-efficient curlers

Magic heating machine

A LITTLE TRICK OF THE EYE

Here's a tip that will make your lashes look volumised. Wash an old mascara brush and roll it through loose setting powder (talc-free baby powder will work too). When the brush is coated, wave the wand through your eyelashes and coat them in powder, making sure that there are no clumps. Then apply your mascara as you usually would for a thick, impressive set of lashes.

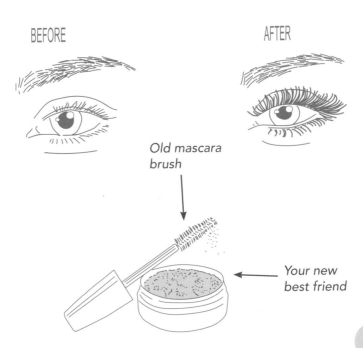

BEFORE

AFTER

Old mascara brush

Your new best friend

MASCARA TIPS

Take your mascara to new lengths by gently drawing the lashes towards the bridge of your nose with three strokes of the brush. Then fan them back outwards another three times. Make sure that every individual lash is coated by using the tip of the brush to paint each one and push them into the right place. Wiggle the wand horizontally across the lower lashes and you are done. Grab your bag and get your day started.

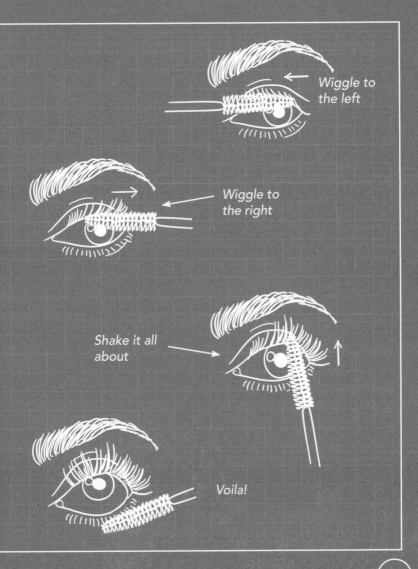

Wiggle to the left

Wiggle to the right

Shake it all about

Voila!

LOYALTY CARD LINER

For perfect liquid eyeliner every time, use a spare plastic credit or loyalty card as a foolproof guide for the elusive perfect 'flick'. Hold the card edge lengthways at an angle, touching your lower eyelid. If you are using eyeshadow too, apply the powder along the card line first and then apply the eyeliner. Starting with the flick, draw along the card. Slowly take it across to the rest of your eye. Was that too easy?

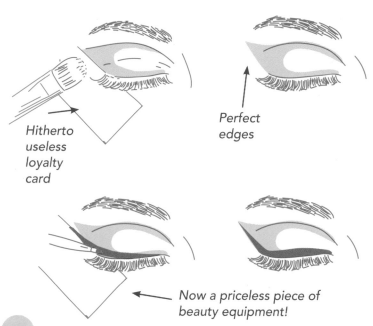

Hitherto useless loyalty card

Perfect edges

Now a priceless piece of beauty equipment!

ELIMINATE MESS

Make your eye make-up look as professional as possible and do away with smudgy streaks across your eyelids with this hack. Simply use a small square of cardboard (a business card is perfect) and hold it behind the lashes as you apply your make-up to create a surface for excess mascara to go onto. You can even cut the card into a curved shape to fit the crescent of your eye.

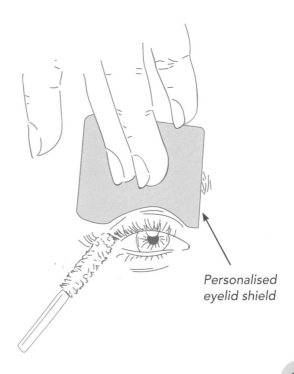

Personalised eyelid shield

ENHANCE YOUR EYE COLOUR

Mix it up a little bit by applying one coat of bright blue mascara to your lashes first. Then brush on a black layer over the top, but leave about a quarter of the blue showing at the lash line. This bright blue ring around the eye will draw the focus to your newly intensified eye colour.

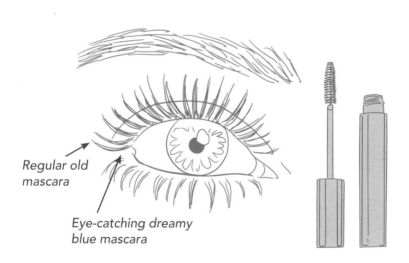

Regular old mascara

Eye-catching dreamy blue mascara

REVIVE OLD MASCARA

Not ready to say goodbye just yet? Here is a tip that will keep your mascara hanging on just that little bit longer. Put a few drops of saline solution – the kind you use for contact lenses – into the mascara bottle, and swill it around to give your slightly gunky mascara a new lease of life.

Old, gunky mascara

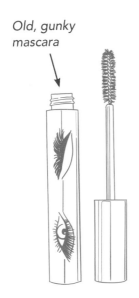

Mascara revitaliser

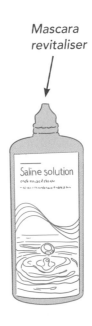

Saline solution

WIDE AWAKE

A pale pink liner will subtly open the eyes to make them look bigger and more youthful. Apply all the way along the bottom of your waterline, as well as in the corners and along the top of the eyelid behind the lashes, to brighten. Another tip: dot and smudge some pink liner underneath your brow to lift and enhance its shape.

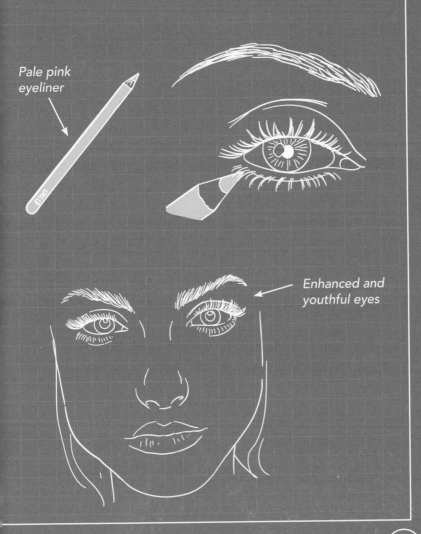

Pale pink eyeliner

Enhanced and youthful eyes

19

CONCEAL A NIGHT OUT

We love the nights out, but not so much the mornings after. If you need a quick fix to look bright-eyed and bushy-tailed, whip out a navy blue mascara to save the day. The dark blue colour does what your black mascara does for your lashes, but it also brightens the whites of your eyes for a much sparkier, awake-looking face – the perfect disguise for faking a good night's sleep!

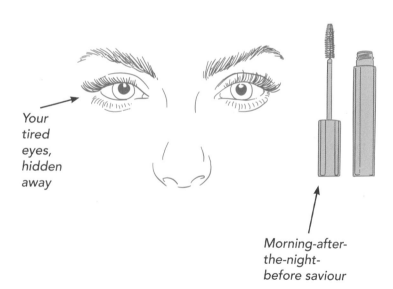

Your tired eyes, hidden away

Morning-after-the-night-before saviour

#SMOKYEYES

Smoky eyes are certainly impressive but achieving them usually takes time and a bit of artistry; two things that are not always on hand! Here is a technique that is infallible and will have you looking like the expert in half the time. Apply a nude or silvery eyeshadow over your lid and then draw a diagonal hashtag in the outer corner with a dark eye pencil or your choice of dark eyeshadow, and blend using your ring fingertip. The hashtag design creates the perfect shape for a smoky eye – and you can layer up the hashtags one at a time for darker looks too.

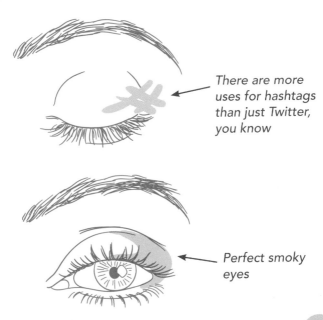

There are more uses for hashtags than just Twitter, you know

Perfect smoky eyes

EMERGENCY LINER

If your eyeliner pencil has rolled away into the unknown or there is nothing left to sharpen, don't panic – your eyes will still look sulky and impulsive when you leave the house today. (This hack is counting on the fact that you still have mascara left!) Use a slim liner brush to take the liquid mascara and apply it along your eyelids. Looking for a smudgy look? Use a charcoal, grey or even brown eyeshadow.

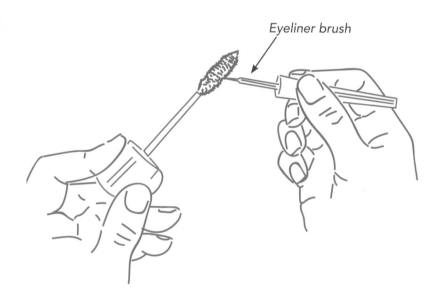

Eyeliner brush

THE LAZY LINER

This is the perfect hack for anyone who is feeling particularly lethargic. Grab your eyelash curlers and effectively kill two birds with one stone. Along the top rim of the curlers, the one that isn't cushioned, draw a line with ordinary, cheapo pencil eyeliner. When the edge is blackened, push them onto your lashes and watch as you curl and line all at the same time – your beauty regime has been halved!

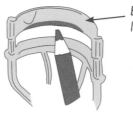

Eyeliner for lazy people

Impressively lined and curled lashes

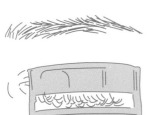
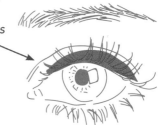

LIGHT-UP EYESHADOW

Sometimes the colour in the pot doesn't look as effective when we actually get around to wearing it. So next time you decide to pull out the sparkly green eyeshadow look, make sure the colours really stand out by covering your lids in bright white eye pencil first. Apply the shadow over the top for a show-stopping look.

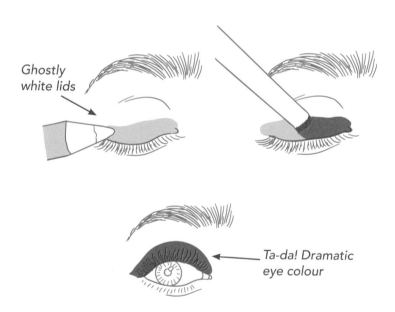

Ghostly white lids

Ta-da! Dramatic eye colour

VASELINE LIP EXFOLIATOR

Flaky lips are a no, so try this for a quick solution. Wash an old mascara brush and get out a tub of Vaseline. Dip the brush into it and gently scrub your lips to exfoliate your pout; flakiness will be gone and lips will be freshly hydrated too.

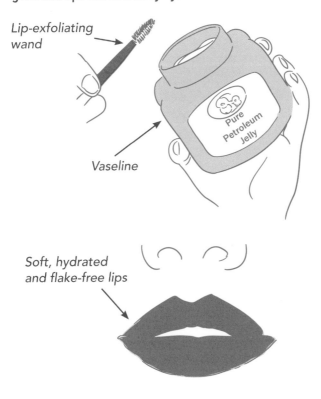

Lip-exfoliating wand

Pure Petroleum Jelly

Vaseline

Soft, hydrated and flake-free lips

A PALETTE CHEAT SHEET

Each eyeshadow palette is slightly different but the principles of how to use the different colours are pretty constant; here are some basic tips so you'll know exactly what you are doing when faced with one. Start with the lightest colour; this will look best as a highlighter just underneath your brow. The second lightest colour goes on your lid and the second darkest colour looks good along the crease of your eye. Finally, the darkest shade should go on your outer corner.

Outer corner

Eyelid

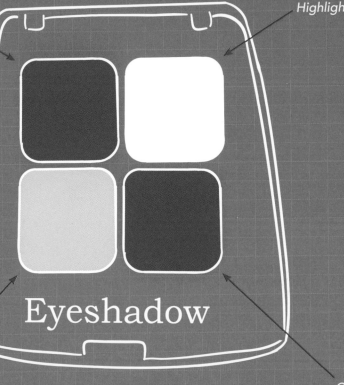

Highlighter

Eyeshadow

Crease

FULLER LIPS

If you want to spend less time on your face and more time out enjoying life – while looking great of course – then try this out. Use peppermint essential oil to plump up your lips. Put a drop of the oil on your fingertip, dab it onto your lips and leave to absorb for 2–3 minutes. Gloss or stick on your lippy for an all-day-long plumper pout.

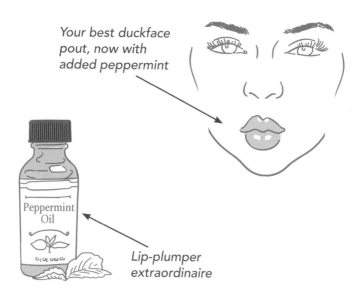

Your best duckface pout, now with added peppermint

Peppermint
Oil

Lip-plumper extraordinaire

3D LIPS

For even plumper lips, here's a little beauty tip to really bring out their fullness. Apply your lip colour and when finished reach for your eyeshadow palette. Choose a metallic light shade – a pink, silver or nude – and use your fingertip to stamp the colour onto the fullest part of your lower lip (the middle). Finish with just a touch in the middle of your upper lip and voilà, voluptuous lips.

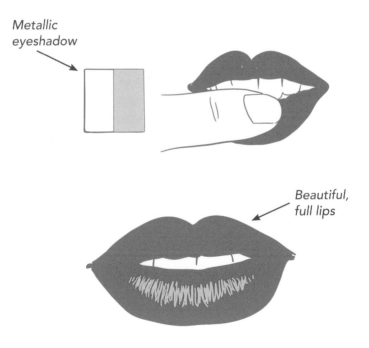

Metallic eyeshadow

Beautiful, full lips

X MARKS THE SPOT

Applying lipstick might seem easy but when you are staring back at yourself in the mirror with red lippy smeared across your chin, you will wonder where it all went wrong. To help, here's a trick for staying in the lines and accentuating the shape of your lips. Cover lips in a layer of concealer or foundation to really make the colour pop. Use a lip liner to draw a diagonal line down from each side of your Cupid's bow to form an X. Starting from the top points of the X, trace around the edge of your lips with the lip liner. Apply the lip colour to the top half of your pout first, using the diagonal lines as a guide. Then apply the rest and get turning heads.

X marks the
Cupid's bow

The perfect
outline for...

Perfectly
filled-in lips

SEAL THE DEAL

To stop your head-turner lips from fading, set them with powder. Simply pull out a thin tissue (separate out a single sheet of three-ply if that's all you have to hand) and lightly hold it across your lips. Dust a few strokes of translucent powder onto the tissue with a brush. Seconds later your lips are sealed!

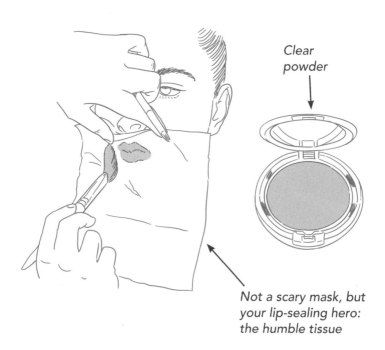

Clear
powder

Not a scary mask, but
your lip-sealing hero:
the humble tissue

MODEL CHEEKS

Ever wondered why models' cheekbones look so utterly amazing? Well, apart from the small matter of a naturally good bone structure, there is a little make-up artistry trick that will really make your cheeks pop. Find the apple of your cheek and apply a circle of blush. Just below the curve of this circle add in a streak of bronzer going diagonally under your cheekbone up towards your ear. Jump down to your jawline and add bronzer all the way along underneath it and finally bronze just above your temple along the hairline. Blend your blush and bronzer with your fingertips; these areas will bring out and define your jawline and cheekbones.

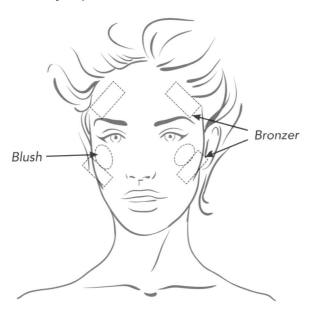

Blush

Bronzer

CONCEALER'S TOP USES

Concealer should be hailed for its versatility, and here are three effects that take seconds to achieve:

1. Use the liquid kind to erase mistakes; if your eyeliner goes skew-whiff just reshape with concealer.
2. If you don't look well rested – pretend! Use concealer to highlight just under the tip of your brow, the middle oval of your eye lid and the inner corner of your eye.
3. Finally, for a natural plump lip, line your lips with it.

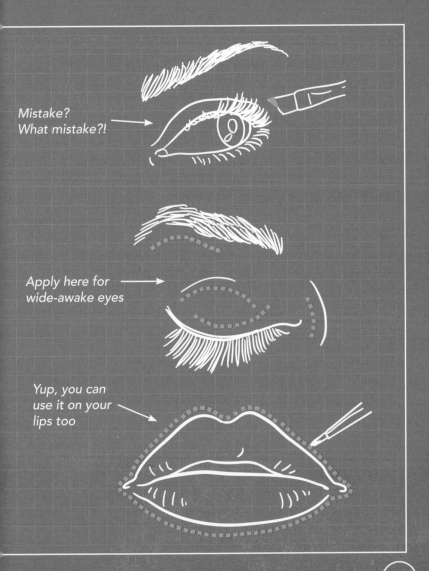

Mistake?
What mistake?!

Apply here for
wide-awake eyes

Yup, you can
use it on your
lips too

COLOUR-CORRECTING LIPPY

Applying red lipstick to your eyes might sound like the kind of idea a toddler would have, but believe it or not, drawing on smudges of red lipstick underneath the eye can really help to conceal dark circles. Apply a light layer under the eye and then put on your concealer as you normally would for long-lasting coverage.

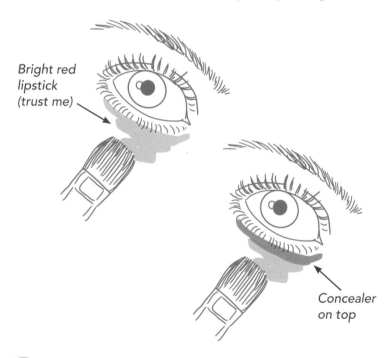

Bright red lipstick (trust me)

Concealer on top

THE PERFECT BROWS

The bold brow is in, but it doesn't need to take long to create. In four easy steps you can have the perfect brows.

1. Brush your eyebrow hair upwards.
2. Define the natural lines of your eyebrows by outlining them with pencil or brow powder.
3. Add thickness and depth with light, upward strokes of your pencil or powder in the natural direction of hair growth.
4. Add in a little highlighter under and above the brows to make them really stand out.

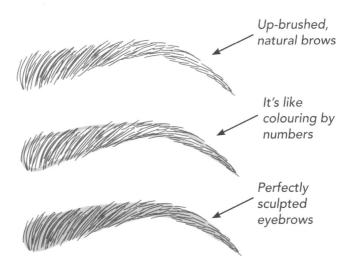

Up-brushed, natural brows

It's like colouring by numbers

Perfectly sculpted eyebrows

ADJUST YOUR BRUSH

Take a blusher brush and turn it into a contouring brush in seconds. Use a hairgrip and slide it down over the hairs of your brush. The clip will hold the brush fibres tightly together, creating the perfect shape to contour with. Get your highlighter out and make your face glow.

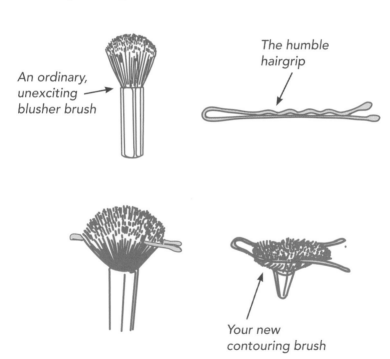

An ordinary, unexciting blusher brush

The humble hairgrip

Your new contouring brush

POWDER REPAIR

Save face and repair your broken powder compact rather than buying a new one, or, worse, doing without! Use rubbing alcohol – the 70 per cent proof kind that you can buy from the chemist – to stick it back together. Cover the compact with clingfilm and use the end of a brush or a spoon to break the powder up into small, even pieces. Add at least 10 drops of alcohol, or enough so that it sticks together, and use a small spatula or the back of a spoon to smooth... just like it never happened!

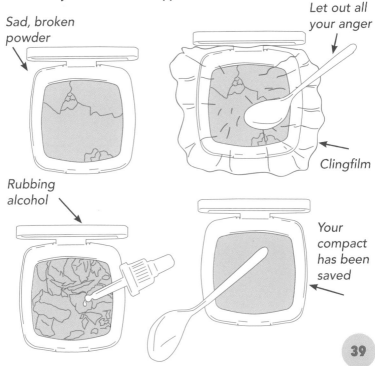

Sad, broken powder

Let out all your anger

Clingfilm

Rubbing alcohol

Your compact has been saved

FRIDGESSENTIALS

Put your essential beauty products in the fridge. OK, the feather boa is just for effect, but seriously, storing your lipstick, nail polish and perfume in the fridge makes them last longer! When your products are exposed to humidity or heat they look and act differently from when you first bought them. Your nail polish can go gloopy, your lipstick sticky and fragrances can even go off. Stash these items in the fridge – yes, next to the pickled onions – and you will enjoy them for longer.

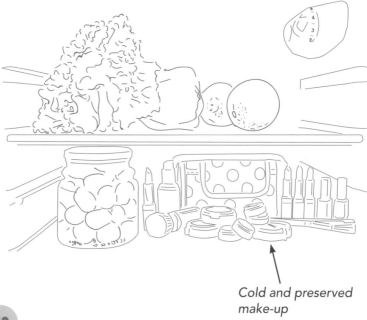

Cold and preserved make-up

MAKE-UP ORGANISER

Throw away your card statements and gas bill reminders – who needs those anyway? – and make way for your new make-up palette organiser. It just so happens that a letter organiser is exactly the right size to hold your bulky eyeshadows, powders and bronzers so they are on display, tidy and lookin' great!

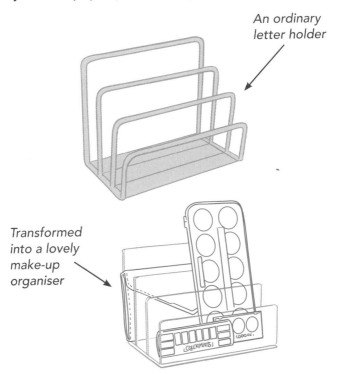

An ordinary letter holder

Transformed into a lovely make-up organiser

SPICED-UP BEAUTY PRODUCTS

Spice up your beauty product storage with a revolving spice rack for a super-easy way to get to your favourite body moisturiser. Simply leave your cooking spices to the professionals and place your revolving spice rack onto your dressing table. Then arrange your favourite beauty bottles on the turn tables for a neat and easy way to store them.

All your goodies to hand

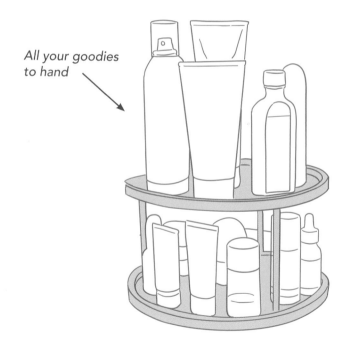

BEAUTY TOOL HOOKS

Get yourself a pack of stick-on door hooks (you can get these from most DIY shops), attach them to the insides of your cupboard doors and hang your beauty tools and appliances on them. Curling tongs, straightening irons, hairdryers and smaller items like eyelash curlers and scissors can be stored on these secret hooks... genius!

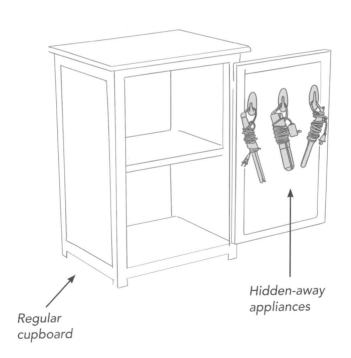

Hidden-away appliances

Regular cupboard

MAKE-UP BRUSH TRAVEL CASE

Going on a trip? Chuck on your coolest shades and put your make-up brushes inside the case. With sunnies perched on your nose you'll be rocking the model look, while your brushes will be kept intact for the duration of the journey, ready for your arrival.

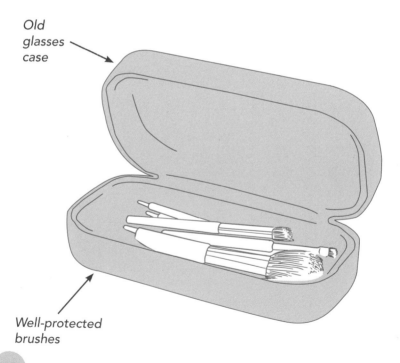

Old glasses case

Well-protected brushes

HAIRSTYLING HACKS

Wouldn't it be a dream to go to sleep and to wake up with perfectly beautiful hair in the morning? A puff of bronzer and a few brushes of a mascara wand and you could be out of the house in no time. Hairstyles don't have to take careful planning and military execution. Flick through this chapter to find infallible techniques that take minutes and will suit you down to the ground.

GET A GRIP

It turns out that we have been using our hairgrips wrong the entire time. Most likely if you have made the effort to use one of these to fix your style in place you have slid the clip into your hair with the raised bumpy side facing up, right? Wrong! To make them grip your hair better turn them upside down. The ridges will attach the clip far more effectively. You can also spray them with hairspray or dry shampoo before using them to give them some extra grip.

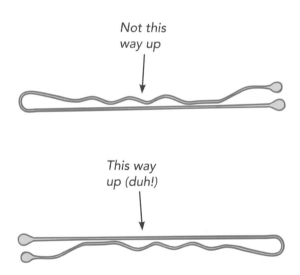

Not this way up

This way up (duh!)

FIGHT FRIZZ WITH SILK

Frizzy, unruly hair is probably one of the last things you want to contend with in the morning, so before your beauty sleep, apply a little serum or leave-in conditioner and bundle all of your hair into a silk scarf, twisting into a turban shape. While the serum is working to soften your hair, the silk is protecting your hair from friction, and thus from frizz, so you can wake up with perfect hair.

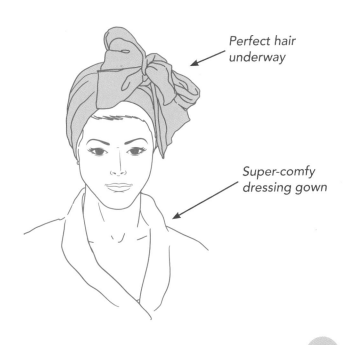

Perfect hair underway

Super-comfy dressing gown

TIE THE KNOT

You will need:
   Scissors
   Lighter
   Ruler
   Dressmaking elastic

Tying up your hair can often result in a strange-looking kink when you take the hair tie out that navigates its way in a horizontal wave right through the middle of your hair. You don't have to spend a fortune to avoid this; instead get busy with some DIY and make your own creaseless hair ties. Measure your flat elastic to size: 25 cm will usually be enough but it does depend on how thick your hair is. Singe the ends with a lighter to prevent fraying, then tie the two ends together and voilà!

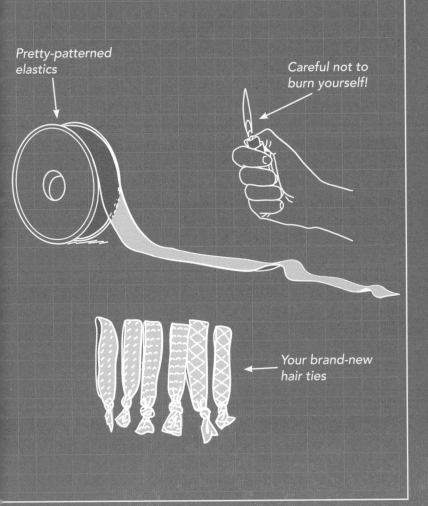

Pretty-patterned elastics

Careful not to burn yourself!

Your brand-new hair ties

NATURAL-LOOKING CURLS

You could of course whip some curling tongs out and spend half an hour or so waving the wand through your hair, perfecting the I-woke-up-like-this wave, but who's got time for that?

First, dampen your hair and then add texturising product for some hold – your curls will last longer this way. (Hint: use the DIY Beach Hair in a Bottle on p.122.) Find your natural parting and split your hair into two halves, then twist each section away from your face. Take your hairdryer and blast each twist with some heat. The result: perfectly natural-looking waves in just 5 minutes.

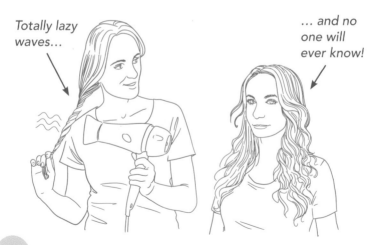

Totally lazy waves…

… and no one will ever know!

MESSY SUPERMODEL WAVES

Supermodels always look pretty cool, even when their hair is sporting a kind of grungy, I-was-born-looking-like-this kind of vibe. So if you fancy looking like you just strutted your way off a moody runway then listen up. Get your straightening irons heating up, then plait your hair in a basic braid and fasten with a hair tie. Bring it round over your shoulder and press the hot straighteners over the plait. When all of your hair has been heated, undo. These imperfect waves look effortless… and they almost are!

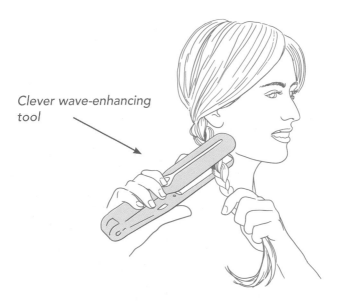

Clever wave-enhancing tool

THE FRENCH TWIST

This is a sophisticated style that looks especially difficult to pull off, but in fact it's actually pretty easy.

Firstly use some salt spray for texture (see p.122) and use the cold setting on your hairdryer to set it. Start at the roots and tease, working your way down to the mid-section. Teasing will help you to mould your hair easily into different shapes. Pull your hair into a mid-height ponytail but don't tie; instead, keeping your hair taut, twist from the ends and start to roll it inwards to the left. Keep rolling until you meet your head and then fasten with hairgrips.

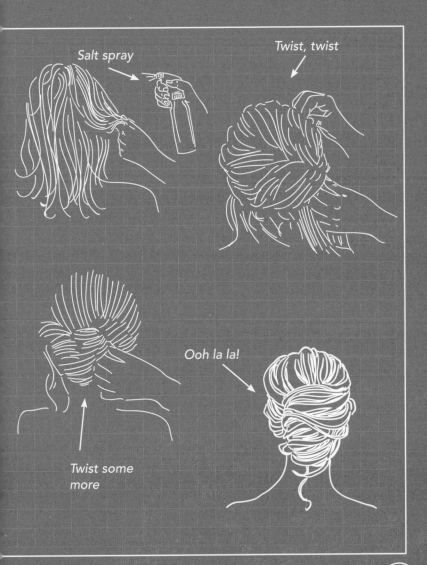

Salt spray

Twist, twist

Twist some more

Ooh la la!

BLURRED LINES

Are your roots giving away the fact that your hair isn't quite as thick as the hot air and backcombing suggest? Simply dust a shade of eyeshadow that is similar to your hair colour along your parting. Shading your hair parting slightly will create an illusion that your hair is super-thick and lustrous.

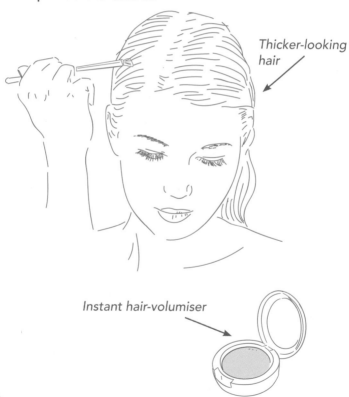

Thicker-looking hair

Instant hair-volumiser

PROP UP YOUR PONYTAIL

Does your ponytail lose its perk as the day wears on? This quick and easy trick will make sure yours stays up high all day. Tie up your hair as you normally would and then insert two hairgrips to the underside, through the elastic and towards your scalp. Fluff up your ponytail and get on with conquering your day.

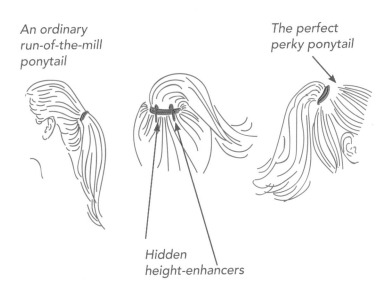

An ordinary run-of-the-mill ponytail

The perfect perky ponytail

Hidden height-enhancers

SLEEPING BEAUTY CURLS

This trick takes around 3 minutes and a night's sleep to achieve your desired look, and all you need is a stretchy hairband. If you haven't got the time to plug in the hairdryer, this hack could be for you.

First lightly dampen your hair and then slip the hairband on. Grab a 5 cm section of hair from the front, lift up towards your face and wrap it into and around the hairband. Repeat this step until all of your hair is tied in small sections into the band. Simply go to sleep and remove in the morning; brush through for bigger waves and finish as you normally would.

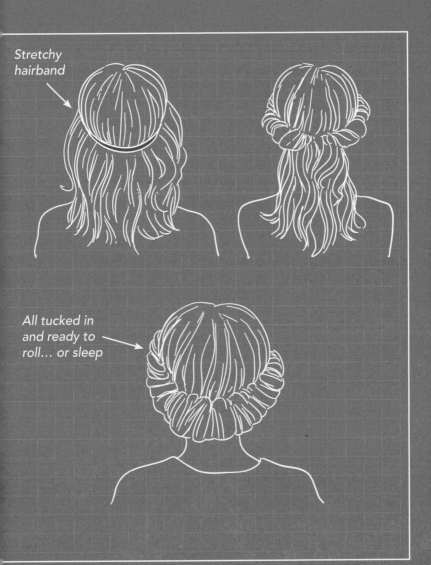

Stretchy
hairband

All tucked in
and ready to
roll... or sleep

THE PERFECT MESSY BUN

Why is it that the messy-look hairstyles usually use the most hair products and take the longest to construct? Well, with these four simple steps you can create a messy bun in no time, without any mind-bending techniques.

1. Tie your hair into a loose, high ponytail. Don't use a brush to tie it back, remember that you are going for the unkempt look.
2. Tease two or three sections of your ponytail using a small comb – this will give you the texture and volume you need.
3. Separate your teased ponytail into two sections and wrap in opposite directions. Secure each with a hair grip.
4. Gently pull on any parts that seem too tight and release a few strands at the front to continue the messy look at the front.

Best of all, your bun will look best with slightly dirty hair, meaning you can press the snooze button on your alarm clock more often! If it is freshly washed apply a little dry shampoo to add texture and grip.

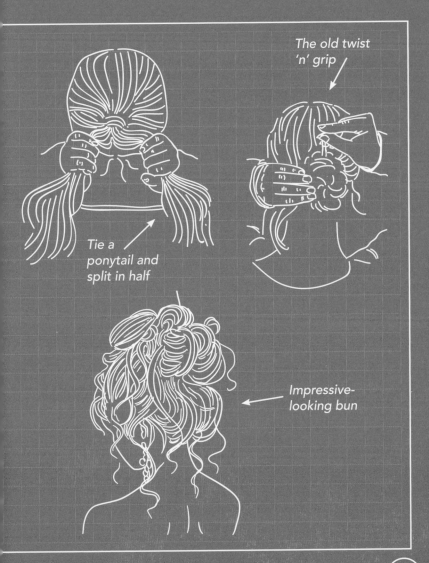

The old twist 'n' grip

Tie a ponytail and split in half

Impressive-looking bun

THE OFFICE LOOK

This style will take you 2 minutes to get right, so it's perfect for the weekday mornings when you would rather spend a few more precious moments under the covers.

Pull your hair into a low ponytail, leaving a few loose strands at the front to frame your face. Part the hair just above your hair tie and make a loose hole with your fingers. Then take your ponytail and thread it through the hole you've just made. Depending on how long your hair is you might be able to thread it through again. Then plait the remainder of your ponytail and fold it in once again. Fasten with a hairgrip.

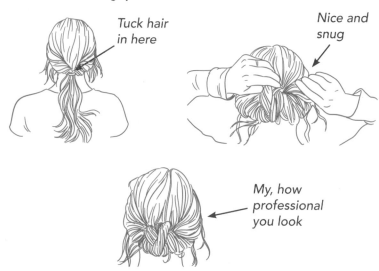

Tuck hair in here

Nice and snug

My, how professional you look

WASH YOUR BRUSHES TOO

Putting dust and oil back into your hair isn't the best recipe for healthy hair. The solution? Wash your brushes; it will take just 10 minutes. Gather up your selection of brushes and combs, clear the hair from them and place them in the sink (leaving wooden ones on the side). Add one teaspoon of shampoo and one teaspoon of baking soda to half a sink of warm water, then use a toothbrush to lightly scrub the bristles and pad. Do the same with wooden brushes without getting the wood parts too wet. Rinse and place them to dry on a towel.

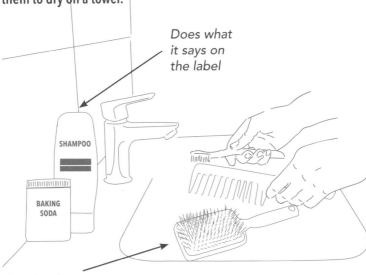

Does what it says on the label

SHAMPOO

BAKING SODA

Lovely, clean brushes

GET TO KNOW YOUR HAIRBRUSHES

Having the perfect selection of brushes will help you to save bags of time when you're getting ready. A purse-sized paddle brush is perfect for the girl-on-the-go, while a larger paddle brush detangles long and thick hair. A small-barrelled bristle brush is for shorter hair types and for smoothing a fringe, while a vented metal bristle is for speed drying while adding a bit of volume and curl. The long and slim comb creates the perfect parting and the afro comb is designed for styling and separating natural curls without damaging them. The teasing brush is a wonder brush for creating lasting volume.

*Purse-sized
paddle brush*

*Larger
paddle brush*

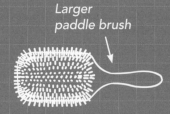

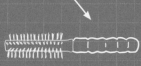

*Small-barrelled
bristle brush*

*Vented metal
bristle brush*

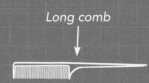

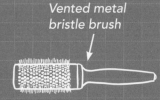

Long comb

Teasing brush

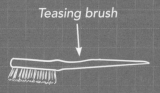

Afro comb

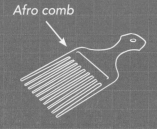

NAIL POLISH TRICKS

How do some girls get perfect nails every time? We might like to believe that they simply have far too much time on their hands and take hours pulling off the flawless polish look, and perhaps they do. Or just maybe they visit the salon twice a week. Don't despair though – it is possible to achieve the same result with the help of these few little secrets. Look like the professionals in half the time!

ROLL, DON'T SHAKE

You might be tempted to shake up your nail polish, but stop right there. Even though this is a popular way of mixing up your colour and preparing your polish it actually isn't the most effective way, as it encourages air bubbles to form, which will muck up your manicure. To prevent this, roll the bottle between your palms for 30 seconds for smooth painting.

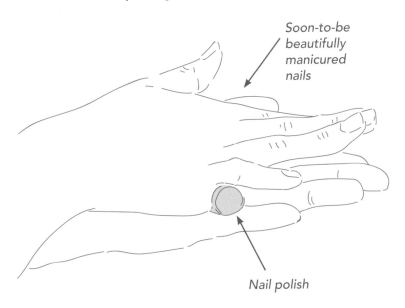

Soon-to-be beautifully manicured nails

Nail polish

THE THREE-STROKE RULE

Three strokes of polish is all you need to get the look. Once you have chosen your colour, dip into the pot and get a good-sized bead of paint on the edge of the brush. The key is to get the polish to do most of the work for you, so start at the base of your nail and gently press the bead down. Pull it down the middle, then to the right and down and finally pull it down to the left. Perfect nails in seconds!

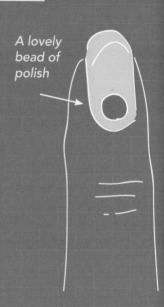

A lovely bead of polish

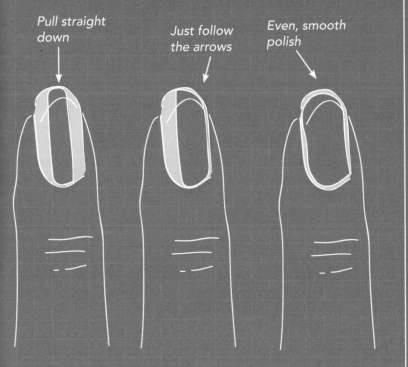

Pull straight
down

Just follow
the arrows

Even, smooth
polish

SMUDGE FIX

If you smudge your perfectly painted nails, this hack will help you to repair the damage. First rub the smudge with a little nail polish remover, either on your fingertip or on a cotton bud. This will smooth the edges of the mark. Then you are ready to paint over it with the same colour, before sealing it with a top coat.

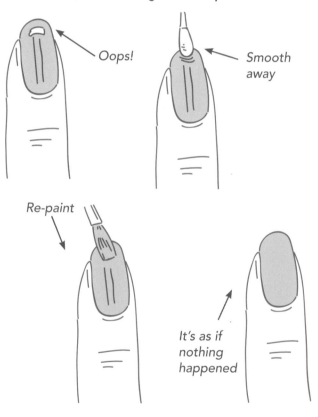

Oops!

Smooth away

Re-paint

It's as if nothing happened

AVOID HOT WATER

Don't dive straight into the shower or bath after doing your nails, even if the warm water erases your I-can't-stop-painting-on-my-skin mistakes, because hot water and nail polish are not friends. The heat causes the nail beds to expand, which forces the paint to stretch with it. This causes cracks and peeling – not a good look for your hands. So always remember to do your nails after you've washed, or at least a couple of hours beforehand to give them time to dry firm.

This may look relaxing, but don't do it!

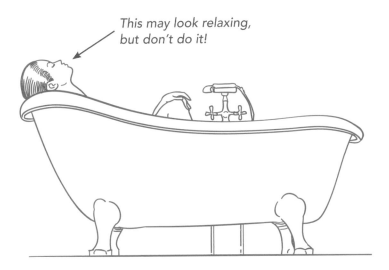

FAST DRYING

Cold water, on the other hand, works wonders... don't jump into a freezing cold bath, though, whatever you do. If you've got to get the day going and fast, don't sit around waiting for your nails to dry, immerse them in cold water or run them under the cold tap for the paint to dry almost instantly.

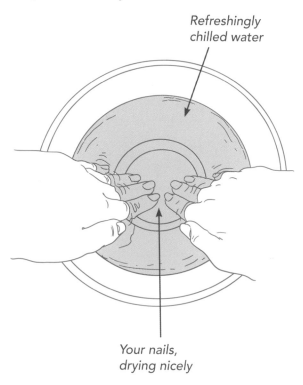

Refreshingly chilled water

Your nails, drying nicely

A FILING MANUAL

This manual only needs a page, it's simple. Sawing away at your nails might make you look the part but moving the file back and forth over each nail will actually tear away at the edge and leave it jagged. Always pull the file across the tip of your nail in one direction only, as filing them the wrong way will lead to broken, peeling and cracked nails – no, thank you.

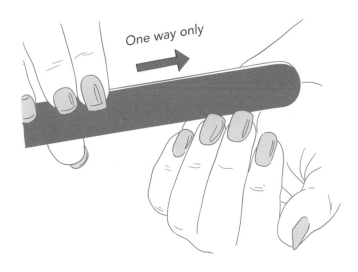

One way only

THE POLISH HOLDER

Do you feel like you need another set of hands to help you paint your nails? The answer lies in the jaws of your hair clip. Find yourself a medium-sized claw clip and stand it up on a flat surface. Open it and place your nail polish pot inside at an angle that is convenient to dip your brush in and out. Close the clip to fasten the pot, unscrew your nail polish and get on with beautifying your fingertips.

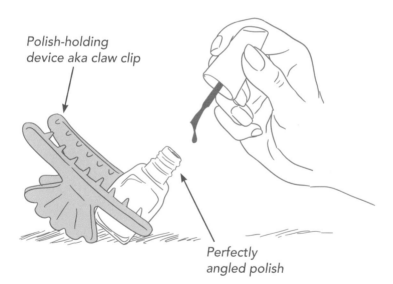

Polish-holding device aka claw clip

Perfectly angled polish

STAY IN THE LINES

If you have trouble staying in the lines, here is an invisible trick that will make sure you get your nail polish perfect every time. Get a cotton bud and dip it into a tub of Vaseline. Apply the Vaseline around the skin closest to your nail. This layer will act as a barrier to the nail colour. Paint as you normally would, mistakes and all, and when the nails are dry you can simply wipe away the Vaseline and any excess paint along with it.

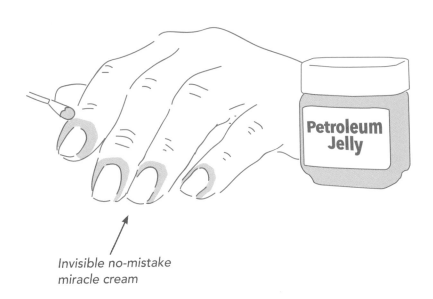

Petroleum Jelly

Invisible no-mistake miracle cream

MASTER THE MANI

The manicure might look simple but we all know it's one of the hardest things to get right. Paying someone to do it will work, but what if you could do it quicker and for free? Get yourself an elastic band and tie a knot into the middle. Put one loop over your thumb and the other around the fingertip you want to paint. Arrange it just below the tip to give you a guideline for the perfect French tip shape.

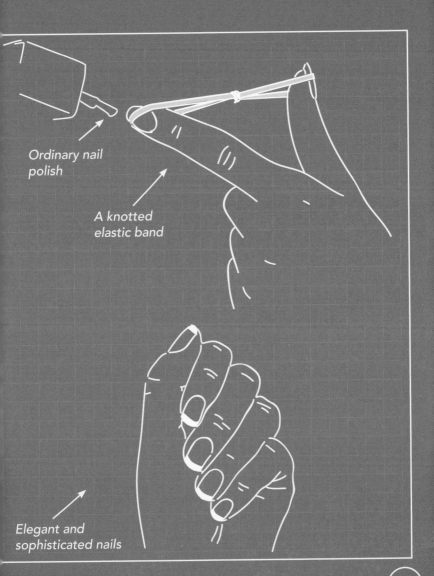

Ordinary nail polish

A knotted elastic band

Elegant and sophisticated nails

MAKE YOUR COLOURS POP

You've found it: the most vibrant shade of summer orange you've ever seen. You might even go so far as to say it's the perfect colour. But often, when you put polish onto your nails, the natural tint of your fingers changes the colour. To get the true shade of the bottle, paint a white layer on before applying your bright summer colour.

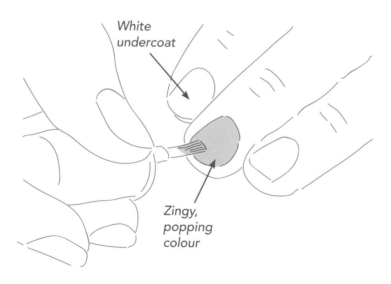

White undercoat

Zingy, popping colour

LONG-LASTING NAILS

To save yourself time and nail paint, apply distilled white vinegar to your nails with a soft cotton pad before brushing on the polish. This might sound like it will just make your hands smell terrible, but trust me, it won't. The white vinegar will dry out the nail surface, removing any residue or moisture that might interfere with your base coat. Your perfect manicure's life has been extended.

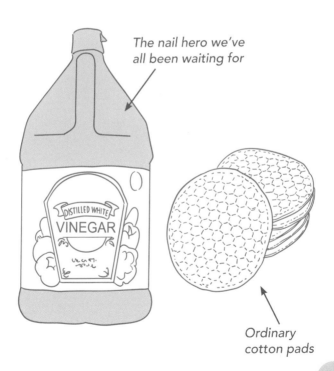

The nail hero we've all been waiting for

DISTILLED WHITE
VINEGAR

Ordinary cotton pads

UP YOUR NAIL TREND

This manicure look will have them believing that you've got it together. The half-moon mani is right on trend and this hack will have you doing it in minutes. Go to the stationery cupboard and dig out some paper hole-reinforcement stickers. After applying a base coat, press down the stickers over the cuticles, covering some of the nail. Paint on polish and when dry remove the stickers. Tidy up the edges with a cotton bud and nail polish remover. Who said nail art was hard?

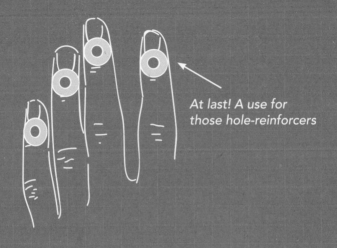

At last! A use for those hole-reinforcers

Jazzy nail art

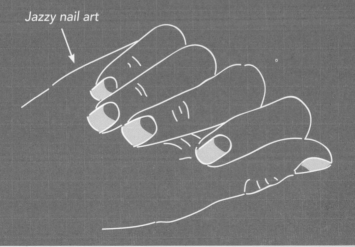

NO-CHIP TIPS

The tips are usually the first to go, so here's how to make sure your base coat protects them. Paint the first layer of the coat to the top half of your nails. Let them dry and paint the second layer of base coat over the entire nail this time. This simple technique will prevent your nails from chipping, making them last even longer.

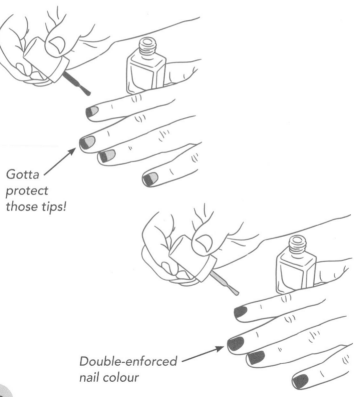

Gotta protect those tips!

Double-enforced nail colour

OMBRE NAILS

Pick three shades for your ombre nails, for example pale blue, bright blue and dark blue. Paint your nails with the lightest shade of polish first and wait for it to dry. Then use an eyeshadow sponge to apply the two other colours: put the bright blue nearest the top of the sponge and the dark blue below, muddying the colours a little where they meet. Press the sponge onto the nail, with the top of the sponge facing your cuticle, and roll it across for the perfect ombre look.

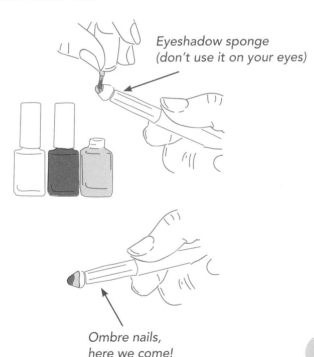

*Eyeshadow sponge
(don't use it on your eyes)*

*Ombre nails,
here we come!*

GLITTER REMOVER

Timeless glitter can suit almost any occasion, any season. Lots of people avoid it because it is an absolute nightmare to get rid of once it's painted on, but there's an easy way to take it off. Soak a cotton pad in nail polish remover, fold it in half and wrap it around your fingertip, securing it with a piece of foil. Repeat this step for all your glittery nails and leave to soak for 5 minutes. Pull off to reveal plain, natural nails.

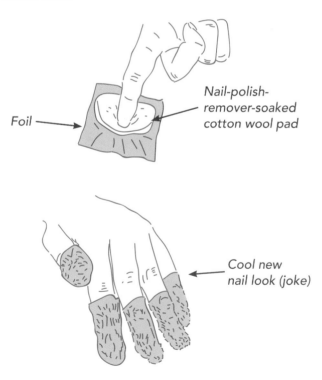

Foil ⟶

Nail-polish-
remover-soaked
cotton wool pad

Cool new
nail look (joke)

GLAMOROUS NAILS

Feel like glamming up with some rhinestones, but struggle to pick the tiny blighters up? Use your brow or eye pencil to pick them up, lift them and then stick them down on your nail. Simply hover over your chosen stone with your pencil, apply a little pressure and when you lift the pencil up, the glittering jewel will be in tow.

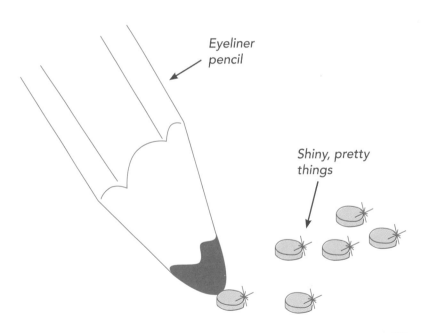

Eyeliner
pencil

Shiny, pretty
things

POLISH REMOVER POT

Make your own nail polish remover pot for an ever-so-lazy way to take off your colour. Fill a small, empty (clean) jar with two small sponges. Push one down to the bottom of the jar. Then take your second sponge, wrap it around a pen (as a guide for your finger) and place it on top of the first. Remove the pen and pour nail polish remover into the jar. Once the sponges have soaked up the liquid, you can place one finger at a time into the sponge to remove your nail polish. Just fasten the lid when you've finished and refill with nail polish remover whenever the sponges dry out.

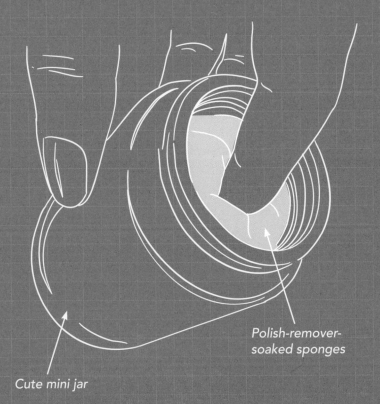

Polish-remover-
soaked sponges

Cute mini jar

POLKA DOTS

Create the perfect, evenly rounded dots with nothing other than a hairgrip. Paint your nails a bright or funky colour and wait for them to dry. Dip your pin into another colour – get creative and pick something wacky – then touch your nail with the pin and lift to create your dots.

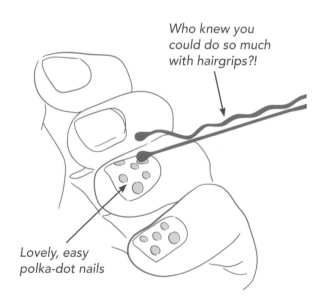

Who knew you could do so much with hairgrips?!

Lovely, easy polka-dot nails

BOTTLE GRIP

Having trouble opening your nail polish? Get a grip! No, really, wrap an elastic band around the lid until it is tight to provide extra grip, so that when you come to paint your nails you won't have a fight on your hands. You could also try rubbing some Vaseline around the lip of the bottle before you close it to prevent any polish from drying the top shut.

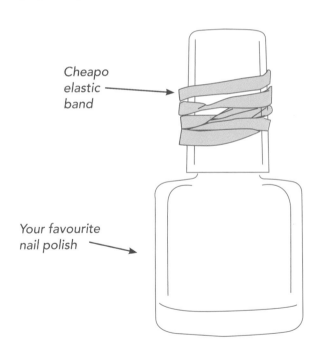

Cheapo elastic band

Your favourite nail polish

SKINCARE: FACE

Somehow the glowing skin you get just after a facial seems an impossible feat to achieve in your own bathroom. Do we really need to play whale music while lying down in a wet Himalayan mud mask, wrapped in banana leaves, to achieve it? This chapter has a few shortcuts up its sleeve for easier, quicker remedies with the same fabulous results - whale music optional.

DARK CIRCLE REMEDY

Under-eye shadows can be a nuisance, and a dead giveaway that you are over-tired or stressed out, so to lessen their appearance mix together a quarter teaspoon of turmeric with one teaspoon of almond oil – if you don't have almond oil replace it with olive oil. Apply the mixture to your under-eye with a clean make-up brush or the back of a teaspoon. Note that this bright spice might stain clothing materials so be very careful when applying it. Leave the mixture on for 20 minutes and then wash away with water. Repeat this three times a week for the best results.

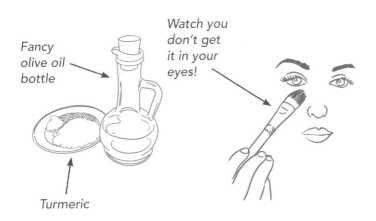

Fancy olive oil bottle

Watch you don't get it in your eyes!

Turmeric

PARSLEY EYE MASK

Parsley contains vitamin C, vitamin K and chlorophyll, which all help to lighten the skin around the eyes and reduce puffiness. Tear off a handful of organic parsley and roughly chop the leaves and place them in a bowl. Crush the leaves as if you were making a cocktail; the back of a wooden spoon is good for this. Then pour two tablespoons of boiling water over the parsley and leave to cool. Use two cotton pads to soak up the liquid and place these over your eyes for 10 minutes.

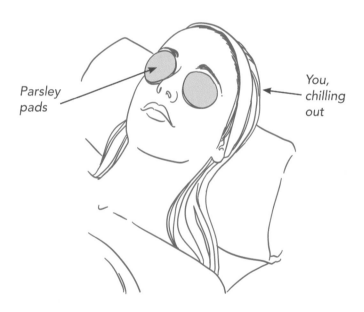

Parsley pads

You, chilling out

A SPARKLING FACIAL

First popularised by Japanese and Korean women, the sparkling water face wash is a tip that many beauticians swear by. The bubbles in carbonated water help to oxygenate skin while purifying and tightening pores, leaving your face looking bright and fresh. To get the glow, pour equal parts sparkling water and still mineral water into a large bowl. You can either dip your face into the water for 10 seconds or use as a toner by applying with a cotton pad. For radiant skin repeat this just once a week.

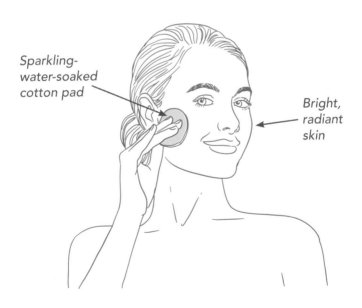

Sparkling-water-soaked cotton pad

Bright, radiant skin

GO GREEN STEAM FACIAL

Green tea is high in antioxidants and even has anti-ageing qualities. It's not all about drinking it either: we can use it on our skin too. Fill your sink with boiling water and then add an organic green tea bag or two; fresh green tea leaves are great to use as well. Reach for a towel, put it over you and bend your head over the basin. Let the steam envelop your face for 3–5 minutes; it will open your pores, allowing hydration and antioxidants to get right into the skin.

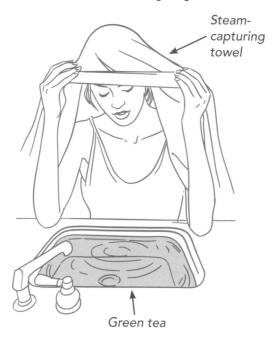

Steam-capturing towel

Green tea

TOMATO FOR BLEMISHES AND SPOTS

Tomatoes are high in vitamins A, C, E, K and B6, which nourish and enrich the skin while helping to close pores and keep skin clear. The acidity in tomatoes helps to reduce and clear up acne – vitamins A and C are also commonly found in many spot treatments sold in shops. Mix together one tablespoon of tomato juice with a few splashes of lemon juice. Apply the mixture to the affected areas and leave for 5 minutes, then wash off. If you want to turn the mixture into a mask, just add natural yoghurt or honey to soothe and hydrate sore skin.

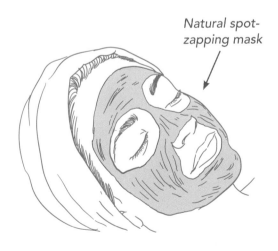

Natural spot-zapping mask

GREEN TEA SCRUB

Exfoliating might sound like a long and unnecessary process, reserved only for those with bags of time, but here is a recipe, filled with antioxidants, vitamins and anti-inflammatories, that takes just 5 minutes.

You will need:
    1 tablespoon powdered matcha green tea
    ½ cup sugar
    1 tablespoon avocado oil

Mix the powdered tea with the sugar to create a gentle exfoliant. Finally stir in the avocado oil for a strong dose of vitamin E. Apply to your skin with your hands and rub in using upward circlular motions. Wash off with warm water.

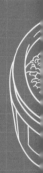

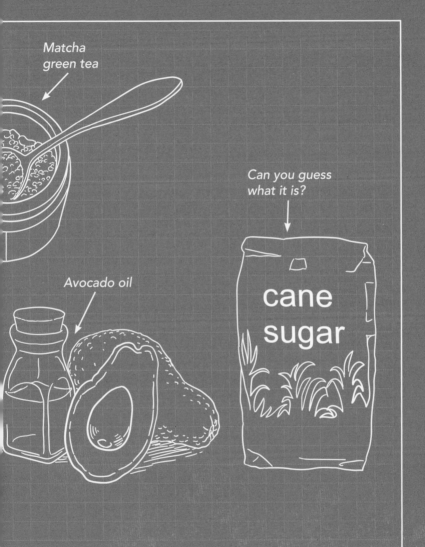

Matcha green tea

Avocado oil

Can you guess what it is?

cane sugar

COCONUT OIL AND GREEN TEA MOISTURISER

To match your exfoliator, here is a recipe for a very green moisturiser: the coconut oil moisturises without clogging pores and the green tea can even reverse sun damage.

Place one cup of coconut oil into a saucepan and put on a low heat to melt. Then add two tablespoons of loose-leaf green tea, cover and simmer for 1 hour. Strain the mixture to separate the tea leaves and whip the coconut oil using a whisk until creamy. Apply this with your hands as often as you would your usual everyday moisturiser and store in an empty moisturiser pot or glass tub. The moisturiser will keep for four to six months.

Magic concoction, simmering away

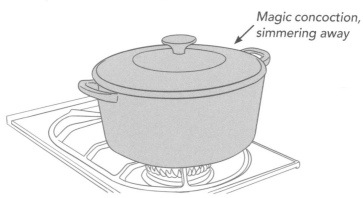

GOLDEN GLOW MASK

Turmeric is what makes this tip golden! This Indian spice slows down cell damage, reduces the appearance of wrinkles and evens skin tone, while also acting as an anti-inflammatory. Also known as the 'Golden Goddess', it has long been used by Indian brides to brighten up their skin before the wedding. Mix together half a teaspoon of turmeric and one tablespoon of coconut oil and apply to your whole face. Leave the mask on for around 20 minutes then rinse away with warm water.

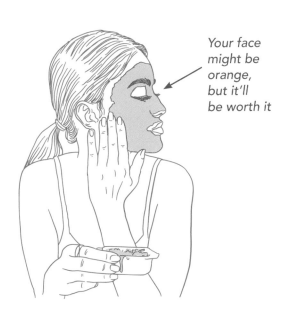

Your face might be orange, but it'll be worth it

AVOCADO AND HONEY FACE MASK

This mask will come to your rescue when you are suffering in the winter months with dry skin. The avocado and coconut oil replenish lost moisture and the honey helps to soothe and heal sore areas. You'll be pleased to know the recipe only requires one half of an avocado… the rest you can eat!

You will need:
- ½ a ripe avocado
- 2 tablespoons honey
- ½ teaspoon coconut oil

Use a blender to purée the avocado until smooth. Then add the honey and coconut oil and mix. Apply the mask to your face, avoiding your eye area, and leave for 10–15 minutes. Remove with warm water.

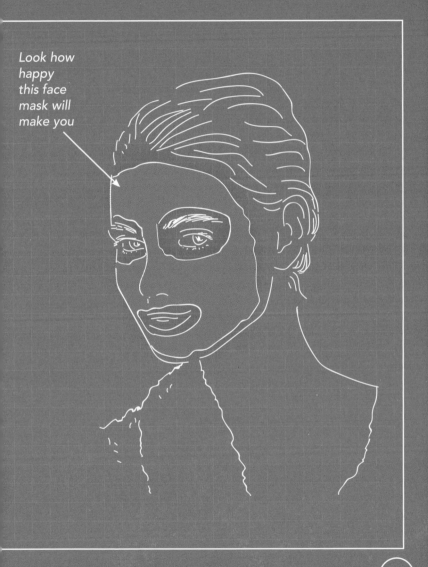

HONEY LIP-PLUMPING SCRUB

You will need:
1 teaspoon honey
1 teaspoon almond oil
Pinch cayenne pepper
2 teaspoons sugar

Mix all the ingredients together in a bowl to form a paste. Rub onto your lips and let the sugar granules do their magic with dry or chapped skin. The honey and almond oil soothe and moisturise, while the cayenne pepper will plump up your lips.

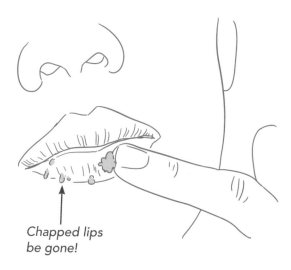

Chapped lips be gone!

EYELASH GROWTH SERUM

Putting on mascara is the extra finishing touch that makes your eyes look wide and beautiful, but what if you want to look wide-eyed and bushy-tailed without make-up? This simple tip is a little care routine for your eyelashes. For long, dark lashes, apply a small amount of olive oil over them with a cotton wool pad or on a clean mascara wand just before you go to sleep. Olive oil is great for hair as it stimulates growth while making lashes soft and healthy. It really is as simple as that.

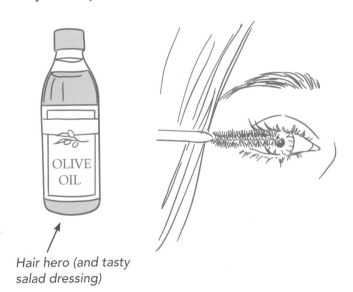

OLIVE OIL

Hair hero (and tasty salad dressing)

BLACKHEAD REMOVAL

Remove blackheads quickly with this simple method. It works best with clean skin, so a good time to try it is after a shower.

You will need:
  Vaseline
  Clingfilm
  A flannel, heated
  Tissue paper

Apply the Vaseline to the affected area and then cover with clingfilm. Place a hot damp flannel over the area to open the pores and press it there for a few minutes. Remove the flannel and clingfilm and use two sheets of tissue paper to cover your forefingers and gently press to clear the pores. Once finished, wash away the Vaseline with water.

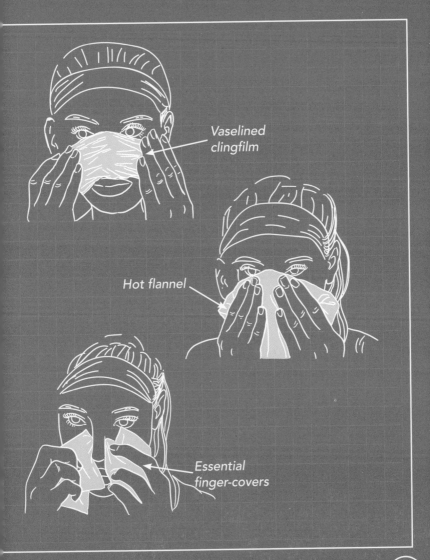

Vaselined clingfilm

Hot flannel

Essential finger-covers

THICKER EYEBROWS

Bushy eyebrows are in and we want them too. Pure pressed castor oil, bought from any health food shop or found online, is a cheap and natural way to grow your brows. The oil contains fatty acids and protein that hair needs to grow long and strong. Before bed, clean your face as usual. Take a cotton bud or an old mascara brush and dip it into the oil. Apply to your eyebrows and use your fingertips to massage it in. Leave the oil overnight, wash it off in the morning and repeat as regularly as you can for the best results.

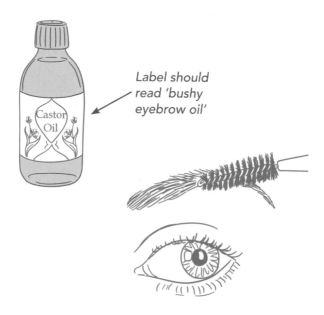

Label should read 'bushy eyebrow oil'

Castor
Oil

YOUNGER-LOOKIN' HONEY

The key to young, dewy-looking skin is moisture. Trendy superfood manuka honey, although rather more expensive than other kinds of honey, might just be the secret beauty ingredient needed for an almost effortless way to great skin. Manuka locks in moisture from the air and holds onto it without making your skin oily. Apply one tablespoon of honey onto clean skin and leave it on like a mask for 20 minutes before washing off. Do this once a week for a supple, youthful glow.

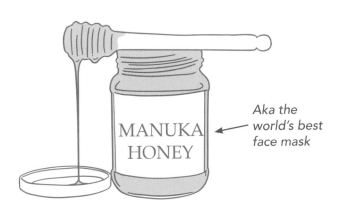

MANUKA HONEY

Aka the world's best face mask

ASIAN BEAUTY WATER

Rice water is one of the oldest and most effective skin treatments in Asia. It cleanses and tones skin with vitamins B1, C and E, and helps to regenerate skin cells and close pores with minerals, zinc and magnesium. Jasmine rice is preferable but if you don't have that, any kind of rice will do. All you have to do is wash half a cup of rice, cover it with mineral water and leave to soak for 2 hours. Strain and keep the water in a dark-coloured bottle. Use this water to wash your skin for a perfect-looking complexion.

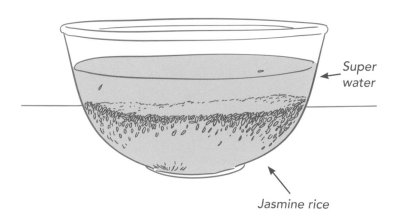

Super water

Jasmine rice

COCONUTTY WHITES

Don't we all want that Hollywood smile, without the bleaching and fancy products? Well, your prayers have been answered with none other than the tropical coconut. Coconut oil pulling is known to reduce the build-up of plaque and is a technique used in the ancient Indian healing practice, Ayurvedic medicine.

To begin, make sure you do this on an empty stomach (it ensures maximum saliva production, making the pulling easier, and is less likely to make you feel nausea), so make it part of your morning routine. Brush and floss your teeth as usual, then swill a teaspoon of coconut oil around your mouth for 5–10 minutes. Spit and rinse your mouth with hot water.

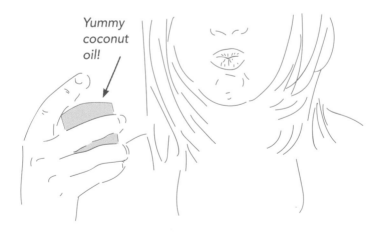

Yummy coconut oil!

STRAWBERRIES FOR WHITER TEETH

Strawberries contain malic acid and vitamin C, which work to remove surface stains caused by wine, tea or coffee, so are perfect to use if you want to whiten your teeth. Mash one to two large strawberries to pulp, stir in half a teaspoon of baking powder and use a toothbrush to apply all over your teeth. Leave to rest for 5 minutes and then rinse off, flossing away any strawberry seeds. Repeat once a week.

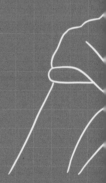

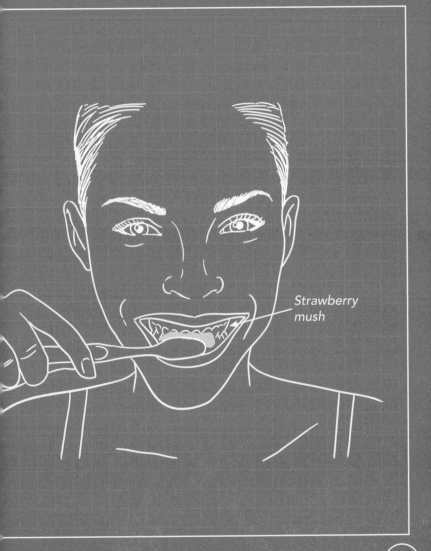

Strawberry mush

SKINCARE: BODY

Typically we focus more on our faces when it comes to skincare, but try not to fall into this trap. The skin on the rest of your body will really benefit from some TLC. There are plenty of tips to try out that will leave you looking and feeling great, and the really brilliant thing is that they won't take you a moment to put together.

BODY BUFF

If you want to buff up your skin naturally while in the shower all you need to do is add a little sea salt to your shower gel. Exfoliating is important if you want your skin to look bright and fresh but rather than going out and buying a separate product, take the au naturel route and exfoliate while you wash. Sea salt is added to many beauty products out there already but you can save your pennies and just add your own – Dead Sea salt is the most beneficial as it also contains minerals that are absorbed into the skin, but regular sea salt will still work wonders.

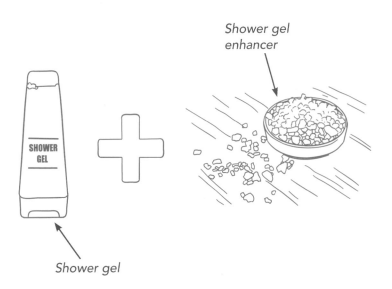

Shower gel enhancer

SHOWER GEL

Shower gel

SUGAR STRETCH-MARK ERASER

Stretch marks are those streaks that can appear on our bodies after rapid changes in growth. Most of us have them but here is a simple treatment that might just make them fade away.

You will need:
1 tablespoon raw sugar
Few drops almond oil
Few drops freshly squeezed lemon

Mix together all the ingredients and rub on for a few minutes every day before your shower and watch those marks disappear.

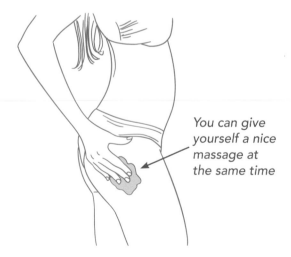

You can give yourself a nice massage at the same time

DON'T WAIT TO HYDRATE

You may have heard that taking hot showers can dehydrate your skin, leading to increased loss of your skin's natural oils. Giving up hot showers might not be the most appealing option, but there's a way around this. Skin contains most moisture when it's wet, and loses it as it dries. The hotter the water the quicker skin cools and the more moisture it loses, so the trick is not to wait around. Moisturise right after a shower. Pat your skin down with a towel and apply moisturiser while your skin is still damp to ensure maximum hydration.

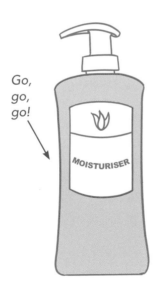

Go, go, go!

MOISTURISER

ISLAND BODY BUTTER

Set aside just 30 minutes to make this body butter and your skin – and purse – will be thanking you for much longer afterwards. Gather your ingredients from any health food shop.

You will need:
  ½ cup mango butter
  1 cup shea butter
  ½ cup almond oil
  25 drops mango essential oil

Create a bain-marie by placing a heatproof glass bowl over a pan of boiling water, making sure the water doesn't touch the bowl. Add the mango and shea butters and allow to melt. Remove the bain-marie from the heat and remove the bowl from the pan. Add the almond and mango oils to the mixture, stirring thoroughly. Chill in the fridge for 20 minutes and then grab a whisk and whip until soft peaks appear. Massage onto skin for a tropical holiday glow. The butter will keep for around four to six months.

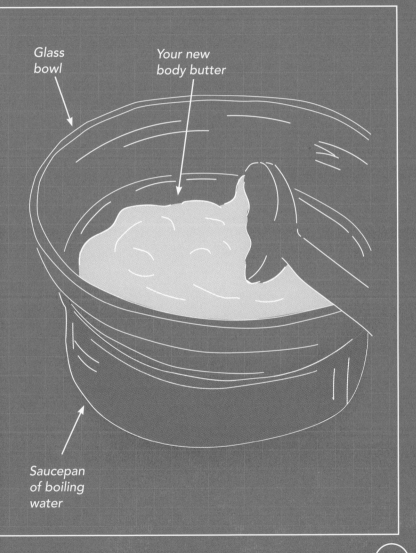

Glass bowl

Your new body butter

Saucepan of boiling water

AVOCADO OIL

If you have particularly dry skin, smooth a bit of avocado oil over your body after moisturising. High in vitamin E and fatty acids, it is a great way to nourish and hydrate your skin. It doesn't take long to reach deep into the skin and has the added bonus of being able to boost collagen synthesis, which means that with regular use skin will become firmer and lifted. Vitamins A, B and E also help to tighten skin.

Buy oil in a bottle and you can just eat this avocado!

A true wonder fruit

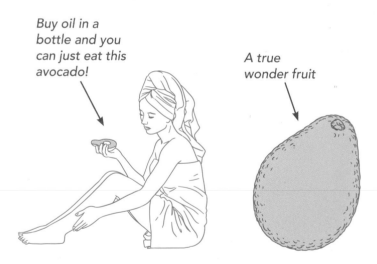

LIME DEODORANT

All out of deodorant? This hack is a quick fix in times of emergency. Keep your limes in the fridge so that they stay cool and then slice one in two. After showering apply the lime straight onto your underarms. Make sure that you haven't recently shaved there, otherwise it might sting! An alternative method is to squeeze the limes and apply the juice with cotton pads. Wait until dry and get on with your day; disaster solved.

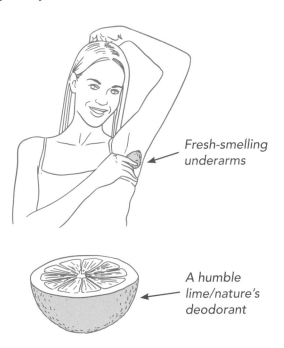

Fresh-smelling underarms

A humble lime/nature's deodorant

WEARING PERFUME

Perfume is an important addition to finish off an outfit, and to get the best out of it make sure you apply your scent in all the right places. Perfume releases its fragrance when skin heats up, so apply it to the areas that are going to get hot: your navel, the small of your back, your chest and the back of your knees, for example. Put on perfume right after a shower before getting dressed, because at this point your skin is most moisturised and able to lock in the most smell.

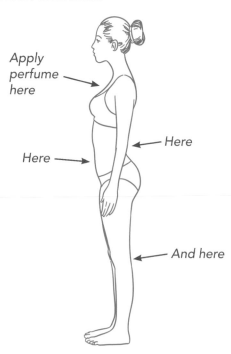

Apply perfume here

Here

Here

And here

PREVENT BLISTERS

Whether you're a ballerina or a 9–5 high heeler, stop blisters in their tracks when you start to feel the pinch. Before you put your shoes on, cover your feet in roll-on antiperspirant for an all-day blister barrier. With this on, your feet won't sweat and without sweat your chance of developing a blister will be very small.

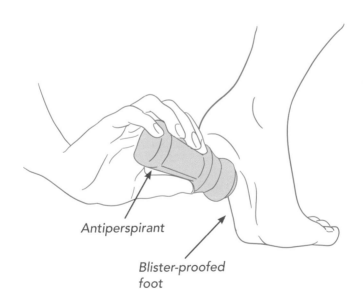

Antiperspirant

Blister-proofed foot

HAIRCARE

Do you long for a straightforward, no-nonsense approach to looking after your hair, but still want to make your mop look fantastic? It's seriously simple with these clever hacks. Whether your hair is curly or straight, short, average length or exceedingly long, there are some simple hacks that will make your haircare routine that little bit easier.

A DE-FRIZZ SERUM

Has your hair naturally got an uncontrollable desire to frizz outwards, even with the slightest breeze? The polysaccharides in aloe vera gel restore your hair's moisture, protecting it from the scourge of the seasons, and for extra frizz-fighting power argan oil will hydrate and give it shine.

You will need:
   1 cup water
   2 tablespoons aloe gel
   1 teaspoon argan oil
   1 teaspoon glycerin
   Spray bottle

Mix the ingredients (all readily available from a good chemist or online) together for a quick and easy solution that you can spritz onto dry or wet hair.

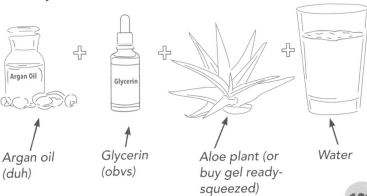

Argan oil
(duh)

Glycerin
(obvs)

Aloe plant (or
buy gel ready-
squeezed)

Water

BEACH HAIR IN A BOTTLE

Achieve the beach bum's ultimate hairstyle with a recipe for salt spray using ingredients you might just have around the house.

You will need:
- 1 teaspoon salt
- 250 ml freshly boiled water
- 1 teaspoon coconut oil
- 1 teaspoon hair gel or conditioner
- Few drops essential oil of your choice (optional)

Dissolve the salt in the water, then add the coconut oil and hair gel or conditioner. You can also add your own signature scent by putting a few drops of scented essential oil into the liquid. Pour the mixture into a bottle with a spritz lid and shake. Wait for it to cool and then spray onto the ends and mid-sections of your hair, and scrunch for a truly windswept look. Now imagine yourself kicking back with a piña colada by the beach – ahh, that's the life.

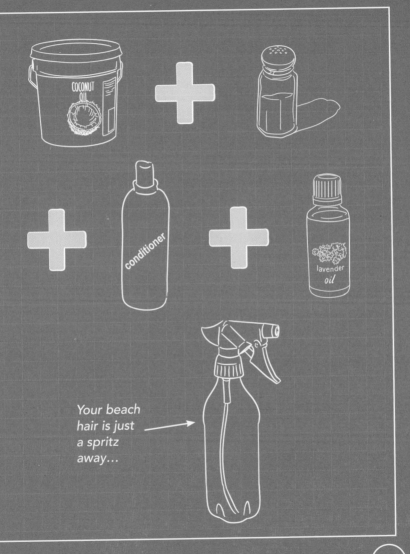

Your beach hair is just a spritz away...

LIGHTEN UP WITH LEMON

UV rays can make blonde hair fade, so before you venture out into the sun spritz on some lightening spray. The citric acid in the lemons will open up the hair cuticles and lift the pigment, while the camomile will really help to lighten the colour, as it contains a plant compound perfect for brightening up blondes – natural or highlighted! Illuminate your locks with this cocktail of all-natural, inexpensive ingredients.

You will need:
  2 cups hot water
  Juice from three lemons
  2 teaspoons almond or coconut oil
  10 drops camomile essential oil

Mix well and pour your ingredients into a spray bottle, remembering to shake with every use.

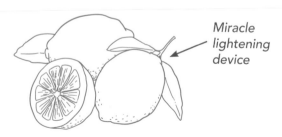

Miracle lightening device

AWAKEN YOUR HAIR

Keep a bottle of aloe vera gel in the shower and when you next wash your hair, add a little to your favourite shampoo and wash as you normally would. The aloe will take your shampoo up a gear and moisturise a dry scalp, preventing those unwanted flakes by keeping your skin hydrated. It's also great for sunburn. Amino acids in the aloe will give your hair strength and shine. Using this powerful plant extract regularly can also promote hair growth as it reduces thinning and rejuvenates hair follicles.

Shampoo enhancer

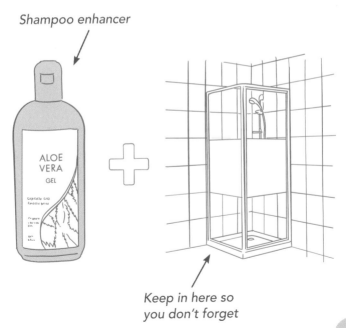

ALOE
VERA
GEL

*Keep in here so
you don't forget*

HAIR REPAIR MASK FOR DRY AND DAMAGED LOCKS

Avocados contain good fats, which are not only good to eat but also benefit your hair by repairing dry and damaged ends. Adding honey to the mask mixture will give your hair strength, while the olive oil will help to hydrate. An optional extra is essential oil, which will smell good and keep dandruff at bay.

You will need:
  1 ripened avocado
  2 tablespoons olive oil
  2 tablespoons honey/agave syrup
  1–3 drops essential oil (optional)

Note: double the ingredients for particularly long or thick hair.
Mix the ingredients well, either in a bowl with a potato masher, or blitz in a food processor. Apply the mask to damp hair and cover with a shower cap. For the mask to really penetrate your hair, use a hairdryer to throw on some heat or sit in the sunshine. Leave your hair for 30–40 minutes, rinse and wash as usual and revel in your soft-to-the-touch tresses.

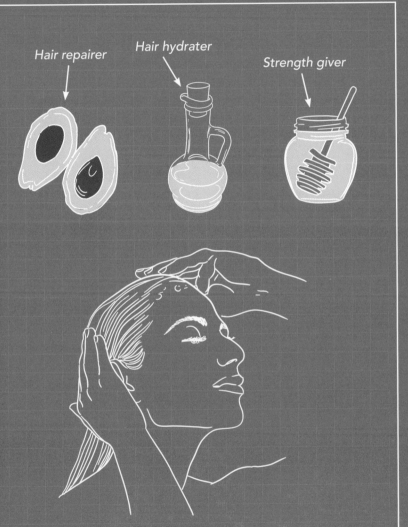

Hair repairer

Hair hydrater

Strength giver

SCENTED HAIRBRUSH

Find a hairbrush with a spongy middle and spray your favourite perfume into it. When it comes to doing your hair, your brush will leave behind a light, sweet scent among your locks. So while you are going about your daily business, you and your hair will smell great! The perfect quick tip that makes a big impact – keep your hairbrush in your handbag to top up your scent during the day.

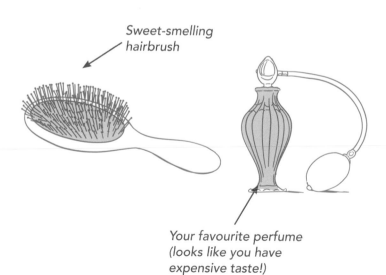

Sweet-smelling hairbrush

Your favourite perfume (looks like you have expensive taste!)

HOME-MADE HAIR PERFUME

Want sweet-smelling locks for a fraction of the price? Is that even a question? Here is a really simple recipe for perfume that won't dry out your mop, leaving it fresh and smelling beautiful.

You will need:
  Spray bottle
  ½ glass distilled water, rose water or witch hazel
  Aloe vera gel or jojoba oil
  5–10 drops of essential oil

Which type of water you go for is completely up to you, and all work equally well. Pour the water of your choice into the empty spray bottle and then add the aloe or jojoba. Finish off with the essential oil. Shake well before each use and spritz into your hairbrush or straight onto your hair. Easy-peasy!

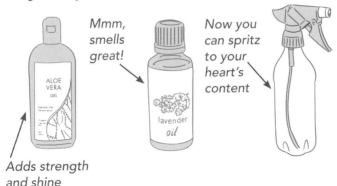

Mmm, smells great!

Now you can spritz to your heart's content

ALOE VERA GEL

lavender *oil*

Adds strength and shine

129

WHIRLWIND DRYING

Dry your hair faster and with no frizz using this handy technique, which is especially effective when drying curls. When hair is wet, it is smooth and defined but when it's dry it can take on a very different look – slightly more on the wild side, shall we say. Believe it or not, towels are often the problem: they absorb too much water from the hair and the harsh fibres agitating each strand through vigorous drying ruffle the hairs' cuticles, causing a frizzy effect when dry.

Instead of a towel use a T-shirt! First apply your styling cream or leave-in conditioner and then bend forward and tie your hair into the T-shirt, twisting it up into a turban shape, tying the sleeves to finish. Leave for 10–20 minutes, depending on your hair type, and either air dry or use a hairdryer and diffuser afterwards.

The T-shirt will absorb moisture fast but without causing frizz; it will also absorb any excess product you have already applied to your hair.

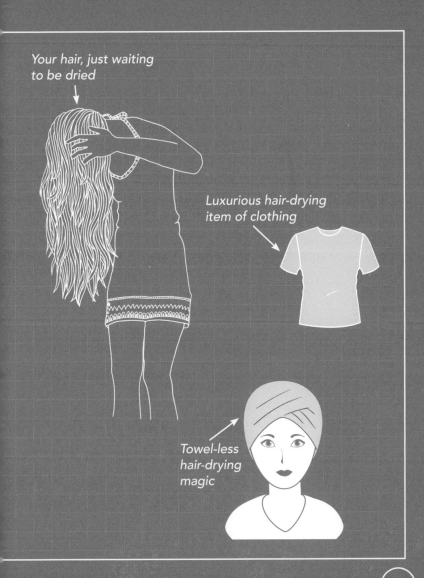

Your hair, just waiting to be dried

Luxurious hair-drying item of clothing

Towel-less hair-drying magic

TAME YOUR FLY-AWAYS

Static is never a great look, but often no matter how much you try to smooth it down, it doesn't seem to make a bit of difference.

A really effective solution is to take a tumble dryer sheet and press it over your hairbrush, through the bristles. As you brush through your locks it will prevent any static getting onto your head. Alternatively, simply brush a dryer sheet over your hair after brushing – it will achieve exactly the same result.

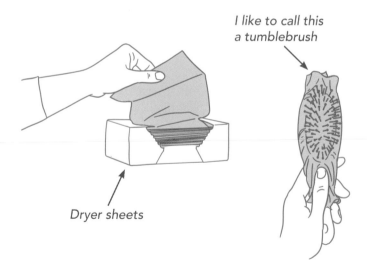

I like to call this a tumblebrush

Dryer sheets

DRY SHAMPOO

Let's face it, we women have a lot on our plates and sometimes we simply have better things to do with our time than wash our hair. Rather than go out and buy yourself cans of dry shampoo, here is a simple recipe that you can put together at home that will achieve the same results.

You will need:
  Empty baby powder bottle
  5–10 drops scented essential oil
  2 tablespoons arrowroot powder
  2 tablespoons cornstarch
  2 tablespoons rice flour
  If you have brown hair, 2 tablespoons cocoa powder

Stir the ingredients through well, then decant into the bottle. Shake onto your roots and rub in with your hands. Brush to blend and style as you normally would.

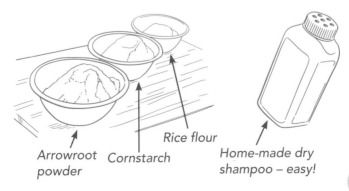

Arrowroot powder   Cornstarch   Rice flour   Home-made dry shampoo – easy!

GOODBYE GREYS

As the stresses and strains of everyday life mount up you may notice that your hair colour pays the ultimate price. A natural way to combat the grey is the application of tea.

You will need:

Black, camomile or red rooibos tea leaves/bags
1 teaspoon salt
Boiling water

Choose the right kind of tea for your hair colour – black for brunettes, camomile for blondes or lighter colours and red rooibos for redheads. Steep your tea in boiling water for 5 minutes. Add salt and stir well. Strain and leave to cool to room temperature. Cover your hair in the tea and massage into the roots. Leave for 30–40 minutes. Rinse but don't wash as shampoo will wash out the natural dyes left by the tea.

Pick your tea wisely (don't drink it afterwards)

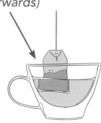

A good excuse for a head massage

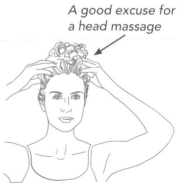

SPLIT ENDS REMEDY

To repair and improve the look of split ends there is a simple, foolproof treatment.

You will need:
   1 tablespoon olive oil
   1 tablespoon honey
   1 large egg yolk
   1 tablespoon coconut oil

Mix together the olive oil and honey. Then add the egg yolk and coconut oil and mix. Apply to your hair, specifically to the ends, and leave for 30 minutes. Rinse and wash out with shampoo. Repeat this fortnightly for a great result. Eggs contain protein and fatty acids as well as vitamins A, D and E, which add moisture and shine to damaged hair. The fatty acids and sulphur in eggs can revive dull hair and provide natural lustre. The egg yolk's rich protein content can also increase hair's volume and make it thicker.

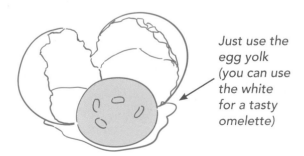

Just use the egg yolk (you can use the white for a tasty omelette)

DEEP CONDITIONING TREATMENT FOR HAIR GROWTH

The key combination for long, healthy hair is strength and moisture. There are a few ingredients to get this balance right.

You will need:
   2 cups aloe vera juice
   1 banana, peeled
   1 avocado, peeled and stoned
   ¼ cup fenugreek powder
   Rice strainer

Fenugreek powder is an Indian spice and the magic ingredient for this recipe. It strengthens and repairs damaged hair while promoting hair growth. Pour the aloe vera juice into a blender, then the banana and avocado followed by the powerful fenugreek spice. Whizz it all up until completely blended and then strain to get rid of any lumps. In 5 minutes you will have yourself a creamy hair miracle-worker. Apply to dry hair and let it work its magic for 30–60 minutes.

All hail aloe

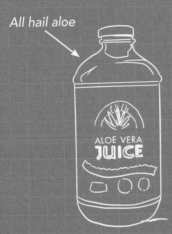

ALOE VERA
JUICE

Yum!

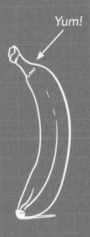

Is there anything
avocados can't do?

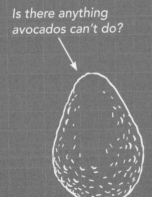

Not-so-secret
ingredient

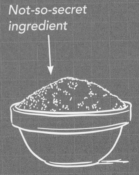

NAIL CARE

Healthy nails are beautiful nails, and with these hacks it really won't take much to keep them looking great.

HOW TO STRENGTHEN NAILS

The broken nail is a lethal fate. To escape this peril simply follow these instructions. Stir in a few drops of freshly squeezed lemon juice to a tablespoon of extra virgin olive oil. Massage into hands and fingernails. Repeat this a couple of times a week and your nails will gradually grow stronger; the lemon juice will stimulate growth too.

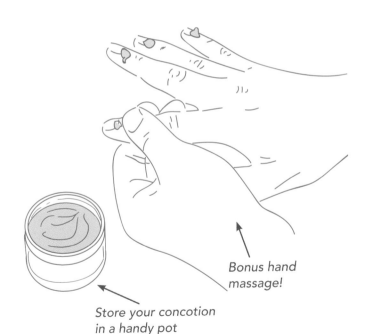

Bonus hand massage!

Store your concotion in a handy pot

NAIL MOISTURISER

Wearing nail colour can really take it out of your nails, and after removing polish you might feel that they are dry and worn out. Try out this nail mask for healthy nails and cuticles. To one teaspoon of olive oil add one teaspoon honey. Mix together and apply to your nails, massaging in around the cuticle area. Leave it on for 10–15 minutes before washing off with warm water.

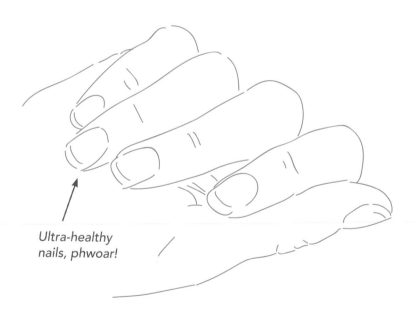

Ultra-healthy nails, phwoar!

CUTICLE OIL

Swiping cuticle oil onto your nail beds is an instant way of looking like you just stepped out of the salon. Looking after your nails doesn't have to be expensive, and in fact you might be able to find just what you are looking for in the kitchen cupboards. Using a cuticle oil on a regular basis does your nails wonders, so delve into the pantry and find a jar of coconut oil. Simply massage a small amount of it into your nail beds, then leave it on to work its magic for 5-7 minutes and wash off.

A cup of tea is the perfect way to while away those 5–7 minutes

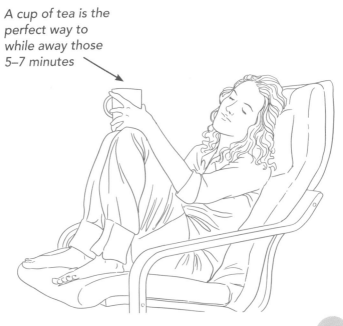

NAIL-BRIGHTENING TREATMENT

Salt is known to soften skin and strengthen nails, while baking soda and lemon lift stains and dullness.

You will need:
- 1 teaspoon salt
- 1 teaspoon freshly squeezed lemon juice
- 1 teaspoon baking powder
- ½ cup warm water

Mix the ingredients together in a bowl big enough to soak both hands. Soak your hands for 10 minutes in the solution and then scrub the fingernails with a soft-bristled brush. Rinse and then moisturise.

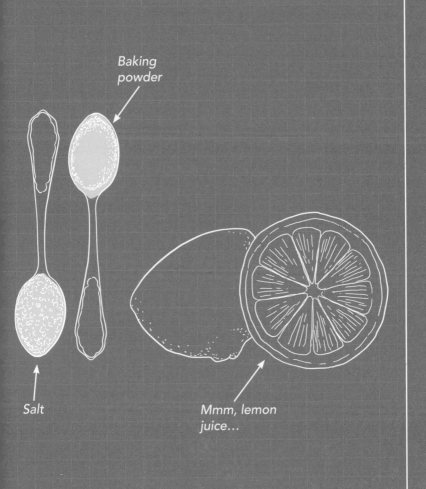

Baking powder

Salt

Mmm, lemon juice...

STUBBORN STAIN REMOVER

If you've been rocking the red nail paint for a while now, you might find that even your nail-polish remover won't get rid of the stains left behind. Go to the bathroom and reach for the toothpaste. Cover your fingertips in paste and gently scrub it in with a brush and warm water. The toothpaste will work away any stains and discolouration for clean and sparkling nails.

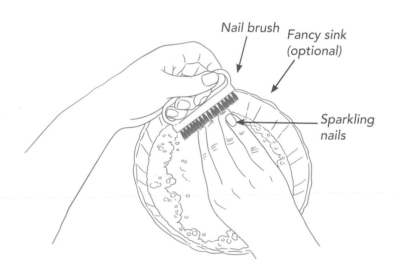

Nail brush

Fancy sink (optional)

Sparkling nails

SILKY-SMOOTH HANDS

Forget about expensive hand creams, here is a recipe for silky-smooth hands to go with your strong, shiny nails.

You will need:
   2 tablespoons coconut oil
   1½ tablespoons honey (raw if possible)
   3 teaspoons salt
   2–3 teaspoons fresh lemon juice

Mix together the honey and coconut oil first and then add the rest of the ingredients, stirring until smooth. Massage a hazelnut-sized amount into your hands for around 2 minutes and then rinse.

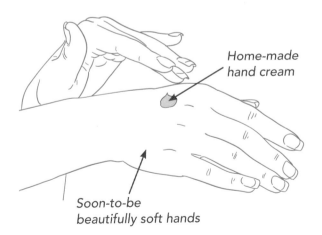

Home-made hand cream

Soon-to-be beautifully soft hands

HEALTHY EATING FOR BETTER SKIN

It is argued that great skin is created from within, so act like a beauty guru and eat your way to beautiful skin. To make it easy, here are some hand-picked fruit and vegetable ideas along with some handy tips for eating and drinking pretty.

GRAFFITI YOUR WATER BOTTLE

Water is said to be the fountain of youth, and we should drink at least eight large glasses of water per day to keep up that all-important hydration. During a busy day it is often easy to forget to drink enough water. To help you remember, mark the hours of the day on a 1-litre water bottle with permanent marker at 200 ml intervals. You'll finish your bottle by noon so then you can refill it for the afternoon. By 6pm you will have consumed eight glasses of water.

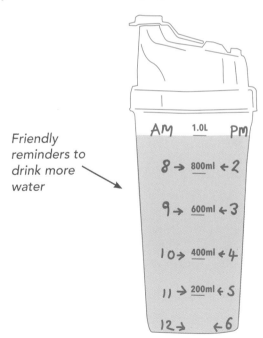

Friendly reminders to drink more water

JUICE FOR PLUMPER SKIN

Dark fruits – black grapes, blueberries, blackcurrants and dark pitted cherries – all contain pigments called anthocyanidins, which are responsible for their dark colour and also act as a powerful antioxidant, and make them perfect for reducing wrinkles. The vitamin C in them also supports elastins and collagen in the skin.

You will need:
   200 ml fresh apple juice
   Large handful black grapes
   Handful blueberries, blackcurrants or dark pitted cherries
   Drizzle olive oil

Put the apple juice in a blender, add the grapes and then the other berries. Blend until smooth. Drizzle in olive oil for a dose of fatty acids to finish.

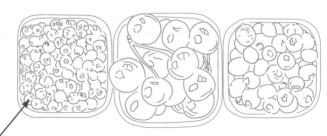

Look at all that delicious fruit!

GLOW LATTE

Fancy swapping out your morning coffee for a golden turmeric latte? It's super-quick to make and does as it says on the tin – it will make your skin glow from within! This spice has pretty much got everything covered: as an anti-inflammatory it reduces redness and dark circles, fights off acne and generally makes your skin bright and luminous while boosting your immune system.

You will need:
1 mug milk (soy, coconut, cashew, almond)
¾ teaspoon turmeric
¼ teaspoon cinnamon
Pinch nutmeg
Honey or agave nectar

Heat the milk in a saucepan and add the spices. Whisk together and add honey or nectar to sweeten. Bring to the boil and continue to whisk. Pour your golden, frothy latte into a mug and drink.

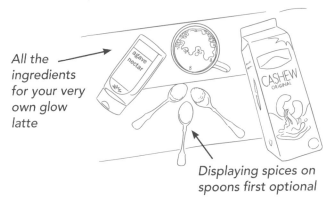

All the ingredients for your very own glow latte

Displaying spices on spoons first optional

CLEARER SKIN SMOOTHIE

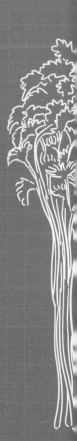

Brighter, more beautiful skin can be achieved with this green smoothie, which both tastes great and makes it easy to get the clear skin you crave. The spinach contains lutein, which makes your eyes sparkle, while a handful of watercress contains more calcium than a glass of milk and is packed full of antioxidants and higher levels of iron even than spinach to help clear those blemishes.

You will need:
   Handful spinach
   Handful watercress
   Handful parsley
   1 pear
   ½ avocado
   Juice of a lime
   4 ice cubes

Blend the fruit and veg until smooth, add ice cubes and sip away.

All these goodies,
about to be
blended up

CLEANSE TEA

If tea is more your thing, then try turmeric steeped in ginger and honey.

You will need:
¼ teaspoon turmeric
¼ teaspoon powdered ginger
Black pepper
Boiling water
1 tablespoon raw, unpasteurised honey

Add boiling water to your ginger, black pepper and turmeric. Stir until dissolved and drizzle in raw honey. Not only will it give you a sweet kick to boost your energy, honey is also packed full of skin-saving antioxidants that help you to regain your natural glow.

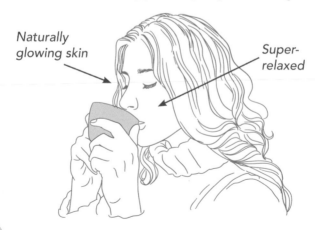

Naturally glowing skin

Super-relaxed

CHOP AND FREEZE SMOOTHIES

Smoothies are a great way to cram in your five-a-day, and five servings of fruit and veg are essential for beautiful skin, but sometimes making time in the morning to prepare a smoothie can be a demanding task, especially when your eyes are closed. So save your fingers, and set aside time at the weekend or one evening after work to portion out, peel and slice your fruit and veg. Put one portion's worth of mixed goodies each into a plastic sandwich bag and freeze for your week's skin-enhancing five-a-day.

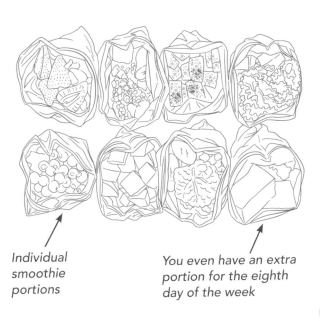

*Individual
smoothie
portions*

*You even have an extra
portion for the eighth
day of the week*

INDULGE YOUR SKIN

Relax and spoil yourself because the great news is chocolate is good for your skin. Dark chocolate, the kind with at least 70 per cent cocoa content, contains flavonols that help your skin to look its best. These are antioxidants that protect your skin from UV damage, meaning fewer wrinkles, and they increase blood flow for a dewy, refreshed look. Eat one 30-g square in the afternoon or after dinner.

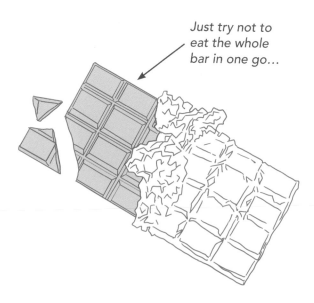

Just try not to eat the whole bar in one go...

IT'S ALL ABOUT WATERMELONS

Drinking water is important but eating it is important for youthful looks too. Watermelons are around 93 per cent water and also contain vitamins A and C, perfect for radiant skin. They make a great snack on their own, or you could try adding it to salads (it goes well with feta and pumpkin seeds) or giving it a spicy twist with black pepper, chilli and a squeeze of lime. Never ignore the seeds; you don't want to miss out on those, as they pack a beneficial punch of antioxidants and fatty acids to keep skin hydrated and fight against break-outs. Roasted watermelon seeds make a great snack – pop them in the oven for 15 minutes at 160 degrees.

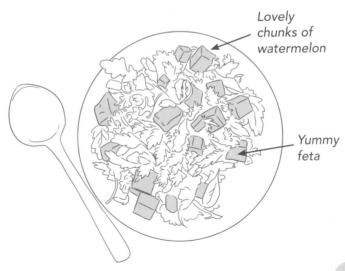

Lovely chunks of watermelon

Yummy feta

BRING OUT THE BEST IN YOUR FOOD

Just bursting with iron

Make your superfoods even more powerful by combining them. Foods that are rich in vitamin C are essential for healthy skin, but an additional benefit is that if you eat vitamin C together with food that is rich in iron, your body can absorb the iron more effectively. Try steaming green vegetables and squeeze a lemon over them, or adding spinach or kale to your dishes as they contain both of these vital nutrients – that way your foods can bring out the best in one another, and not just in terms of taste.

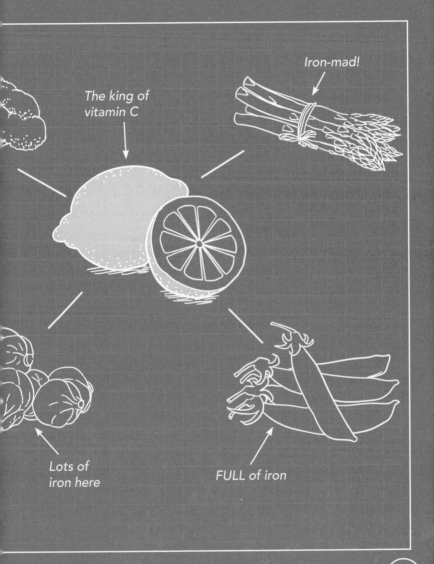

Iron-mad!

The king of vitamin C

Lots of iron here

FULL of iron

157

JAZZ-UP YOUR WATER

Give your water a lift by adding beauty food to your glass. Slice one lemon or lime for a dose of vitamin C and dice a handful of watermelon into small cubes or blend. Add these to 1 litre of water in a jug with around 15 fresh mint leaves and a handful of ice cubes to finish. Leave in the fridge overnight to allow the flavours to steep. Switch your wake-up drink from murky brown tea or coffee to this refreshingly colourful tonic.

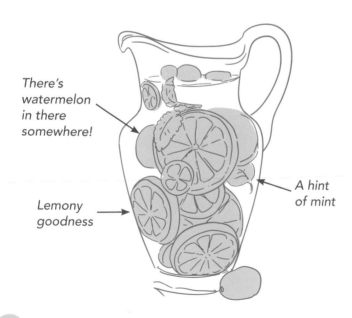

There's watermelon in there somewhere!

A hint of mint

Lemony goodness

BRIGHTEN UP WITH LEMONS

Lemon juice is a cleanser: it helps to flush out toxins in the body, so that your skin will appear brighter and clearer. Wake up and refresh your morning by adding boiling water to a mug with a few slices of lemon (to taste); squeeze in some honey or syrup for a dose of sweetness, or ginger or cayenne for some extra zing, and begin your day feeling bright. A word of warning: the acidity of the lemon can be damaging to your teeth, so it's best to drink your hot lemon through a straw (be careful not to burn your mouth!) so that it bypasses your teeth.

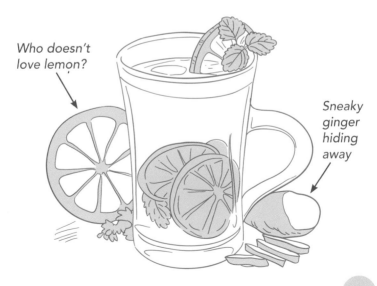

Who doesn't love lemon?

Sneaky ginger hiding away

SLEEP EASIER

Get the beauty sleep you deserve by eating a couple of kiwis before bed. There is a relationship between eating antioxidant-rich foods and sleep: research suggests that eating kiwi fruit before bed may have dramatic benefits for sleep and in a study those who consumed antioxidant- and serotonin-rich food, like kiwi fruit, on a daily basis, experienced a better quality of sleep. Harness the power of the little green furry fruit.

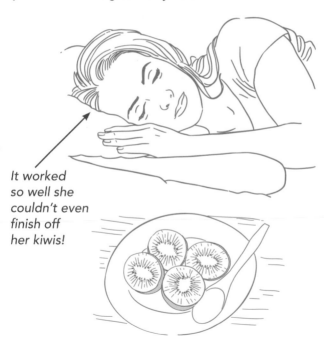

It worked so well she couldn't even finish off her kiwis!

HEALTHY EATING FOR BETTER HAIR

Luscious locks demand nourishment – not just from the haircare products we put on them, but from the food that we put inside our bodies too – so eat beautiful! Here are a selection of hacks to make it easy. Your hair will be down to your ankles in no time.

A SMOOTHIE FOR LONGER HAIR

Sweet potato contains vitamin A, which hair needs for a healthy scalp and to create oils to stop drying and breakage of the hair strands to promote strength and the all-important length. Here's an easy way to get it into your diet, which also gives you a boost of other nutrients that'll help you on your way to sleek, long tresses.

You will need:
  1 banana, peeled
  2 cups almond milk
  Roasted sweet potato, peeled

Blend the banana, almond milk and sweet potato together in a food processor. Aim to drink one of these smoothies a few times a week for best results.

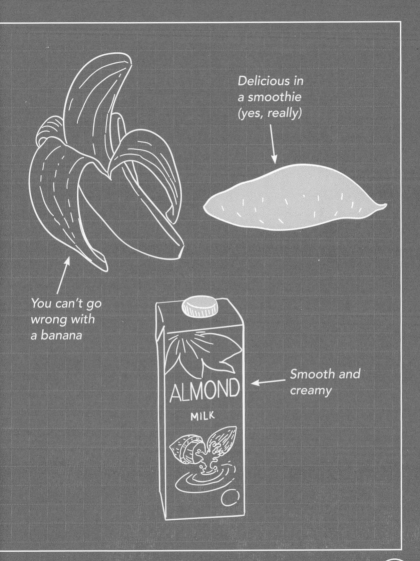

Delicious in a smoothie (yes, really)

You can't go wrong with a banana

ALMOND MILK

Smooth and creamy

GO GREEK

Greek yogurt is a low-fat dairy option that will add a little more protein to your diet, which is perfect for healthy, long hair. It contains vitamin B5, which is also found in many hair products on the market, and vitamin D, which helps the absorption of calcium and hair growth. Dollop it onto granola and red berries with honey on top for a healthy hair breakfast, or freeze it for an after-dinner treat.

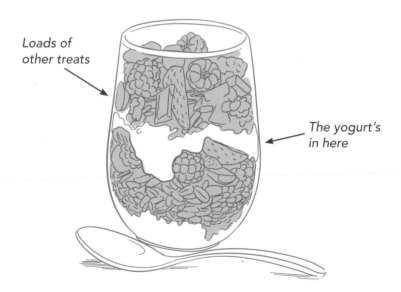

Loads of other treats

The yogurt's in here

HOLYMOLE, WHAT'S YOUR SECRET?

The secret's avocados. Know that, while you are enjoying your Mexican, an extra helping of guacamole might just make your hair shine. Avocados contain omega-3 fatty acids, which keep your hair and scalp hydrated. Our bodies don't naturally produce omega-3s so adding avocado to your diet, especially in the form of a delicious dip, is a great idea and your hair will love you for it.

As if you needed an excuse for chips 'n' dips

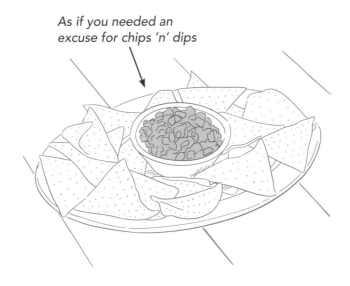

ZING UP WITH ZINC

Hair (even including our eyelashes) relies upon doses of zinc for growth. When we don't get enough of the mineral our hair can shed, so for healthy, full locks indulge in a date with a plate full of oysters and a sprinkle of lemon juice. If oysters aren't your thing then look for other foods rich in zinc - lean beef, spinach, pumpkin seeds, cashew nuts and fortified breakfast cereal are but a few.

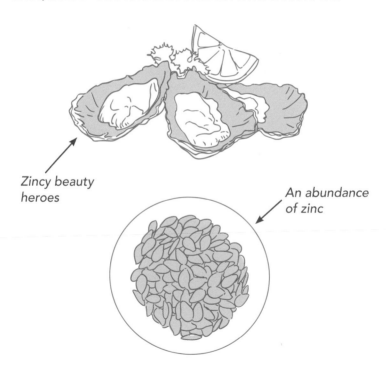

Zincy beauty heroes

An abundance of zinc

EXERCISE

Even a girl on the go needs a few beautifying exercise hacks and tips to sprinkle in over the week. Exercise changes how our skin looks and feels, boosts our circulation and fills our mind with positive, energy boosting endorphins… smiles tend to be a good look too.

JUMP ROPE

Skipping is the ultimate busy-girl's exercise. It's high intensity and, believe it or not, a full body work-out too. Luckily for us, according to the British Rope Skipping Association, 10 minutes of skipping can have the same benefits for our health as a 45-minute run. Once you've purchased your rope you can skip for free just about anywhere and it improves muscle tone, balance, flexibility, heart rate and blood pressure. Try setting yourself a challenge, such as to skip through all the ad breaks of your favourite show, or to your top three mood-boosting songs in the morning to get your day off to an energised start.

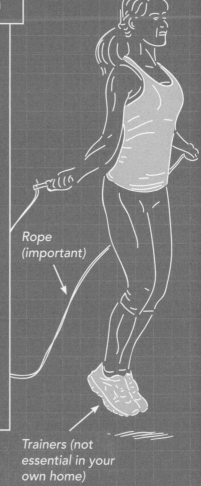

Rope
(important)

Trainers (not
essential in your
own home)

Something wildly
thrilling on TV

LISTEN TO MUSIC

While you skip, plié and downward dog, press play on the stereo and put on your favourite upbeat tracks. Studies show that a distraction such as music can improve athletic performance by 15 per cent, as you are less aware of your exertion. Music itself encourages you to move and the beat even sets the pace, so power through your workout with the positive energy gained from listening to your best playlist.

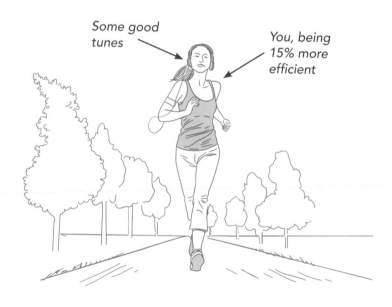

Some good tunes

You, being 15% more efficient

SPOT CHECK YOUR WORKOUT

Take good care of your skin while you work out! Exercising is of course great for our bodies and it's great for opening up pores. So make sure that your face is make-up free, as a combination of sweat and make-up can cause an excess amount of oil. This oil will block pores and can lead to an outbreak of pimples – disaster! Keep cleansing wipes in your gym bag and even if you aren't wearing make-up, cleanse before a workout; be sure to wash your face after exercising too.

It's like this pocket was made for cleansing wipes

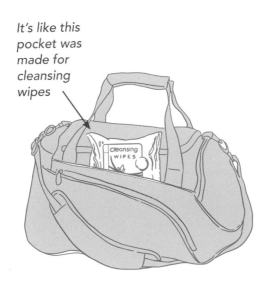

EMBRACE YOUR INNER BALLERINA

Nothing says elegance quite like ballet does, and you don't need to be a professional to get some dancers' moves into your exercise routine. Use heel raises in your warm-up routine, and try this to strengthen thighs, glutes, ankles and feet. Stand, feet together, holding onto the back of a chair for balance. Press up with the balls of your feet, then bend into a deep 'plié' by lowering your hips, keeping your knees touching. With your legs still bent raise up again and repeat 20 times. Try squeezing in some pliés while waiting for the kettle to boil, or while you brush your teeth.

173

HAVE DIRECTION

Set yourself a goal whenever you are getting ready for a workout. Take a few minutes in the changing room or in the car to review your progress and set out in your head what you are aiming to achieve from today, whether it's striving to nail your eagle pose or do one more squat than usual. Having a specific purpose will boost your focus and make sure you get the most out it.

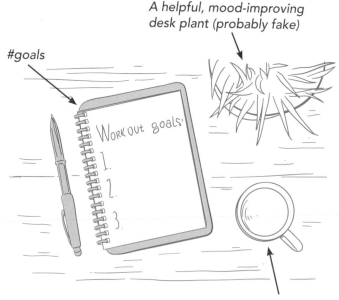

A helpful, mood-improving desk plant (probably fake)

#goals

One of the healthy drinks in this book, I'm sure

PAMPER YOURSELF

Pampering yourself doesn't have to involve going to your local spa and forking out on expensive treatments. Create your own blissful sanctuary right at home for next to nothing. Even if your bathroom has seen better days, there's nothing a candle and some whale music can't fix.

SPA SOUNDS

First things first, get the whale music sorted. Grab your smartphone and use its worldly powers to scan the web for the perfect playlist. There are plenty of waterfall soundtracks, singing mammals and rainforest sounds out there for you to get just the right atmosphere in your bathroom. Remember, though, that breaking your phone via water damage won't be relaxing, so place it in a resealable sandwich bag while you spend time in your new spa.

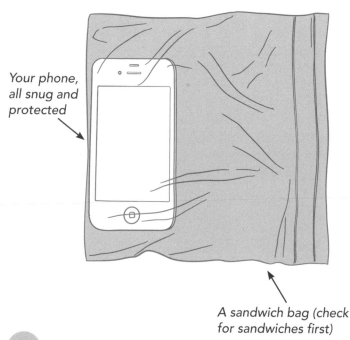

*Your phone,
all snug and
protected*

*A sandwich bag (check
for sandwiches first)*

A GREEN TEA SOAK

For a health- and beauty-boosting treat, add 6–10 green tea bags to your bath. This might sound strange, but you'll be pleased to know that an emerald tea-infused bath can benefit your skin and your well-being in a number of ways. It soothes stressed skin while detoxifying, delays the effects of ageing, helps to repair sun damage and even improves a dry scalp and dandruff (and don't worry, you won't turn green). Not so strange after all… well maybe a bit.

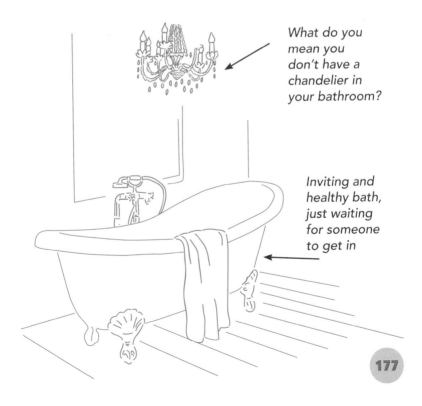

What do you mean you don't have a chandelier in your bathroom?

Inviting and healthy bath, just waiting for someone to get in

CUCUMBER EYE GEL

Soaking in a bath is the perfect opportunity to multitask – peacefully and without any effort, of course. This should be a 'here's one you made earlier' moment when you reach out for the cucumber eye gel pot on the side and slather it on to reduce tired and puffy eyes. It's really simple to make: blend half a large peeled cucumber until it's liquid and then strain, keeping the juice. Add two to three tablespoons of cucumber juice to six to eight tablespoons of aloe vera gel and whisk to mix. Pour into a small jar and leave it to set for 1 hour in the fridge. Use to your heart's content; it will keep in the fridge for six weeks.

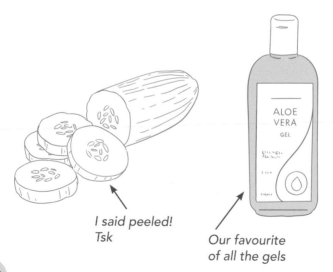

I said peeled!
Tsk

Our favourite
of all the gels

SOOTHE STRESSED EYES

If you haven't had time to create a cooling cucumber eye gel then try this option with yet more tea. Camomile is a natural anti-inflammatory that will ease red and puffy eyes. Steep two tea bags in boiling water for about 3–4 minutes, squeeze out the excess water and then place the bags into the fridge for them to cool. Place the cooled tea bags over your eyes for 15 minutes: when you take them off, your eyes will feel rejuvenated.

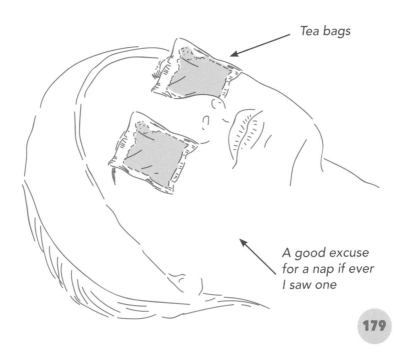

Tea bags

A good excuse for a nap if ever I saw one

STRAWBERRY FEET

Glowing, soothed feet don't take much to achieve, so treat those toes with this sumptuous summer foot scrub.

You will need:
  8-10 ripened strawberries
  2 tablespoons almond oil
  1 teaspoon sea salt
  1 tablespoon vitamin E oil

Blend the strawberries to form a thick, smooth paste. Transfer the paste into a bowl and add the almond oil, then stir in the vitamin E and sea salt. Massage the scrub into your feet with both hands for 5-10 minutes and rinse for soft, beautiful feet.

Beautifully smoothed feet

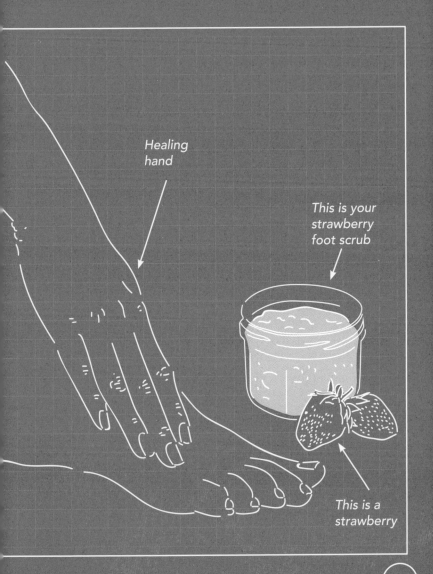

Healing hand

This is your strawberry foot scrub

This is a strawberry

HEAT IT UP

To make it so close to the real thing that you might almost forget you are at home, heat up your body and face lotion. It's a simple and yet effective touch to enhance your spa day and all you need to do is put some of your moisturising cream into a microwavable bowl and heat it up for no more than 30 seconds. Check the temperature, leave to cool if it's too hot, and then apply to your skin for a truly spa-like experience.

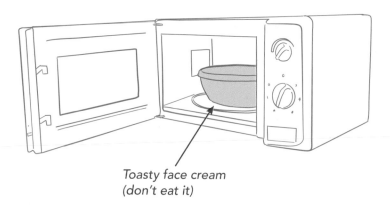

*Toasty face cream
(don't eat it)*

SALT FOOT BATH

If you've been on the go all day and your feet need some down time, make yourself a quick and easy salt bath. Salt is the perfect thing to heal tired and swollen feet and when added to water it makes a high-concentration solution that allows excess water to escape from your feet through osmosis (rewind back to your science days), reducing the swelling. Flick on the kettle and fill a large bowl that will fit your feet. Allow the water to cool to your desired temperature and add half a cup of Epsom or sea salt before plunging your tired feet in for a refreshing lift. Leave your feet in the water for as long as you need – too long, though, and they'll come out looking like well-seasoned sultanas!

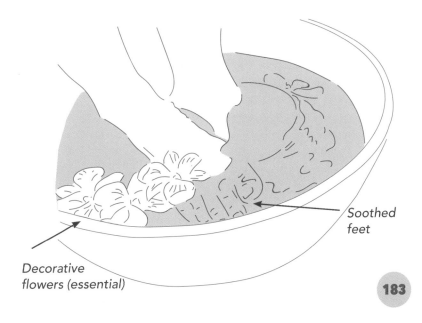

Soothed feet

Decorative flowers (essential)

BEAUTIFUL BODY SCRUB

Polish and revive your skin with a blueberry and lemon body scrub. Silky smooth skin is just moments away with a super quick how-to.

You will need:
- 1½ tablespoons frozen blueberries
- ½ cup coconut oil
- 1 cup sugar (white or brown)
- 1 teaspoon lemon juice or a few drops of lemon essential oil

Break down the frozen blueberries in a food processor and then add the lemon, sugar and coconut oil. Blend for a few seconds and it's ready to go. Your body scrub is best applied in the shower. Massage all over your body and after a few minutes wash away. Exfoliating is best done two to three times a week – a little less for sensitive skin.

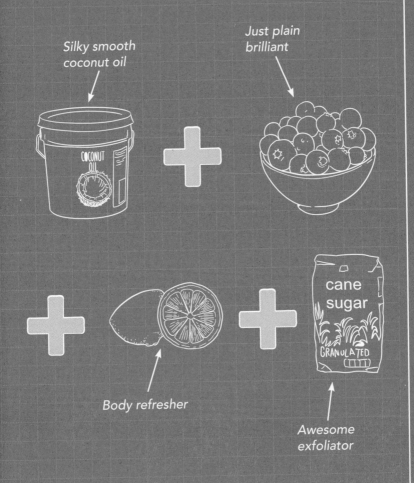

Silky smooth coconut oil

Just plain brilliant

Body refresher

Awesome exfoliator

HOT FACE TOWELS

The star of any facial is the luxurious, steaming hot towel you press on your face for the ultimate indulgence. The great news is that this is indulgent for your skin too, helping to fight off the seasons, keeping skin radiant and healthy. First cover your towel or flannel with an oil of your choice. Coconut oil helps to ward off break-outs; other suggestions are peppermint oil, vapo rub, lavender oil or mango oil. Then either dampen and microwave for 30 seconds or cover with boiling water and ring out. In both cases make sure the towel cools before wrapping it around your face (leaving your nose clear for breathing purposes) for a soothing, spa-like treatment.

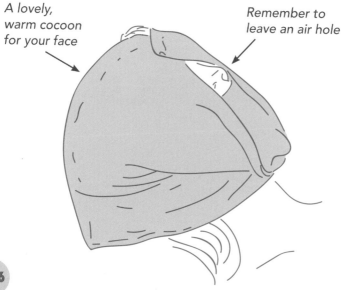

A lovely, warm cocoon for your face

Remember to leave an air hole

ICE CUBES

No spa is complete without cool water to keep you hydrated, but don't just get a glass of tap water, whip up something special instead that tastes great too. Freeze your favourite flavours into ice cubes and add them to your water for a boost of natural goodness. The night before a spa day, fill up your ice cube trays with edible flowers or mint leaves, wedges of lime, slices of lemon or strawberry and cover in water before putting into the freezer. If your trays are too small for slices of fruit, just put sliced fruit straight into the freezer.

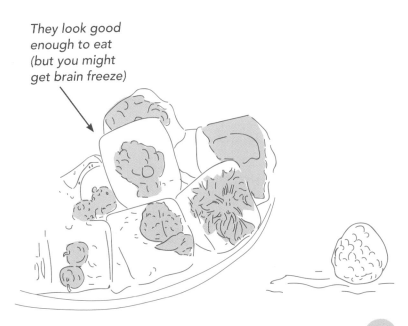

They look good enough to eat (but you might get brain freeze)

FINAL WORD

Congratulations – you are officially a Beauty Hacks champion. Now that you're taking weekly spas at home, cat flicking your eyes to sheer perfection and have your pout puckered up, you've got all the time in the world to get on with doing the fun stuff.

Pass on these jewels of wisdom to all those you meet, and plugging the book wouldn't hurt either.

If you have some hacks that are not featured in this book and think they deserve to be, email them to auntie@summersdale.com.

Until next time – keep beauty hacking!

HACKS INDEX

BEAUTY HACKS

HACKS INDEX

If you're interested in finding out more about
our books, find us on Facebook at
Summersdale Publishers
and follow us on Twitter at
@Summersdale.

WWW.SUMMERSDALE.COM

IMAGE CREDITS